DIVIDED STAFFS, DIVIDED SELVES

Divided staffs, divided selves

A case approach
to mental health ethics

STANLEY JOEL REISER
HAROLD J. BURSZTAJN
PAUL S. APPELBAUM
AND
THOMAS G. GUTHEIL

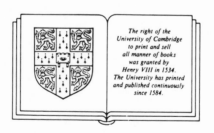

The right of the
University of Cambridge
to print and sell
all manner of books
was granted by
Henry VIII in 1534.
The University has printed
and published continuously
since 1584.

CAMBRIDGE UNIVERSITY PRESS

CAMBRIDGE
NEW YORK   NEW ROCHELLE   MELBOURNE   SYDNEY

Published by the Press Syndicate of the University of Cambridge
The Pitt Building, Trumpington Street, Cambridge CB2 1RP
32 East 57th Street, New York, NY 10022, USA
10 Stamford Road, Oakleigh, Melbourne 3166, Australia

First published 1987

Printed in the United States of America

Library of Congress Cataloging-in-Publication Data
Divided staffs, divided selves.
Bibliography; p.
Includes index.
1. Psychiatric ethics – Case studies.   2. Psychotherapy
ethics – Case studies.   I. Reiser, Stanley Joel.
RC455.2.E8D58   1987   174'.2   86–28416

British Library Cataloguing in Publication Data
Divided staffs, divided selves : a case
approach to mental health ethics.
1. Psychiatric ethics
I. Reiser, Stanley Joel
174'.2   RC455.2.E8

ISBN 0 521 26846 X hard covers
ISBN 0 521 31890 4 paperback

CONTENTS

Contents

ACKNOWLEDGMENTS

THE AUTHORS are indebted to Loren H. Roth, M.D., M.P.H., Director of the Law and Psychiatry Program and Professor of Psychiatry at the Western Psychiatric Institute and Clinic, University of Pittsburgh, for sharing several of the case examples with us. We also acknowledge the help of Archie Brodsky and Leslie Levi of the Program in Psychiatry and Law at the Massachusetts Mental Health Center in Boston and Ruth Anna Putnam of the Department of Philosophy at Wellesley College, who read and commented on different parts of this book. We wish to thank our patients, mentors, colleagues, students, friends, and families, who continue to be our teachers. Among these, Bonnie Cummins a research associate is named as a co-author of one of the chapters. In her acknowledgment, all the chapters and cases deserve to be so coauthored.

ABOUT THE AUTHORS

Stanley Joel Reiser, M.D., Ph.D., is the Griff T. Ross Professor of Humanities and Technology in Health Care at the University of Texas Health Science Center at Houston. In his writing, he has focused on the ethical foundations of health care, most particularly examining the relationship between practitioners and patients, and on the effects of technology in shaping the experiences of patient care and the institutions concerned with giving it.

As co-director of the Harvard Interfaculty Program on Medical Ethics from 1971–82, Dr. Reiser helped initiate one of the earliest teaching and research efforts in medical ethics in the United States. It was in the context of this program that the authors of this book met and began working together. The anthology *Ethics in Medicine: Historical Perspectives and Contemporary Concerns* (MIT Press, 1977), which Dr. Reiser co-edited, was the first comprehensive anthology to appear on this subject. His interest in the consequences of a technological medicine was first expressed in his book *Medicine and the Reign of Technology* (Cambridge University Press, 1978), which explored the effects of an increasing technologic presence in the process of diagnosing illness. He has been a leading figure in the development of the *International Journal of Technology Assessment in Health Care* begun in 1985, of which he is co-editor, and of the society bearing the same name.

At the University of Texas Health Science Center Dr. Reiser co-directs a joint graduate program in health care ethics with Rice University, where he is an Adjunct Professor of Religious Studies and spends a great deal of time doing ethics rounds with students and faculty.

Harold J. Bursztajn, M.D., is co-director of the Program in Psychiatry and the Law and Assistant Clinical Professor of Psychiatry at Harvard Medical School. He has published an extensive body of work in ethics, medical decision making, the doctor–patient relationship, risk management, and malpractice prevention. He has continued to maintain a clinical practice and teaches on both the undergraduate and postgraduate levels.

In *Medical Choices, Medical Chances: How Patients, Families, and Physicians Can Cope with Uncertainty* (Delacorte, 1981) he described the vicissitudes of the doctor–patient sharing of uncertainty throughout the human life cycle. He has pioneered, with other health professionals, in bringing psychoanalytically informed clinical experience into a dialogue with ethicists, medical historians, and social and experimental psychologists. From these collaborations there has grown a body of conceptual and empirical research on the doctor–patient decision-making relationship. He is now exploring the use of image and metaphor to chart, communicate, and resolve ethically, legally, and clinically conflictual areas of practice.

Paul S. Appelbaum, M.D., is the A.F. Zeleznik Professor of Psychiatry and Director, Law and Psychiatry Program, University of Massachusetts Medical Center. His research interests focus on the effects of legal regulation of medical and mental health care and on ethical problems that arise in clinical practice. As chair of the American Psychiatric Association's Commission on Judicial Action, he has helped shape organized psychiatry's responses to the major legal issues of the day. Dr. Appelbaum maintains an active clinical practice and frequently consults with other clinicians on problems of clinical, legal, and ethical concern.

Thomas G. Gutheil, M.D., a graduate of Harvard College and Harvard Medical School, is currently Director of Medical Student Training and co-director of the Program in Psychiatry and the Law, Massachusetts Mental Health Center. He is also Associate Professor of Psychiatry, Harvard Medical School; Visiting Lecturer, Harvard Law School; Lecturer in Psychiatry, Tufts Medical School; President, Law and Psychiatry Resource Center; and Affiliate Member, Boston Psychoanalytic Society and Institute. Dr. Gutheil served as an American Psychiatric Association delegate to the American Bar Association's Task Force on the Insanity Defense. A board-certified forensic psychiatrist, he co-authored, with Paul S. Appelbaum, M.D., the *Clinical Handbook of Psychiatry and the Law* (McGraw-Hill, 1982), which received the 1982 Manfred S. Guttmacher Award as the outstanding contribution to the forensic psychiatric literature. A second Guttmacher award was given to *Psychiatric Uses of Seclusion and Restraint* (APA Press, 1984, K. Tardiff, M.D., editor), to which Dr. Gutheil contributed several chapters.

1

INTRODUCTION

WHEN A THERAPIST and a patient meet to address the needs created by mental disorder, their developing relationship is bounded by rules that determine the appropriateness of interventions considered and performed. These rules are based not only on knowledge about the biological and psychological bases of disorder, but also on values which, like the therapies that can be employed, not only provide a range of alternatives, but also set limits on actions.

This book is about a particular subset of values dealing with ethics. Ethics is a discipline concerned with understanding the right-making and wrong-making characteristics of actions. The practitioners who analyze the ethical dimensions of human thought and interaction must examine deeply held beliefs derived from personal experience concerning right and wrong, cultural mores founded on the conventions of tradition, values received from and embodied in decisions of courts and legislatures, historical conventions developed by the health care professions over time and embodied in documents such as ethical codes, and scholarly works on ethics.

In this book, we approach ethics through case studies. Our goal is to present case material that can provide clinicians with a basis for learning and reflection, preferably in interaction with their colleagues. The cases used are real and are derived from clinical situations and consultative experiences of the authors, and their colleagues. The use of the case method, as applied to problems of mental illness, was developed by the authors at the Massachusetts Mental Health Center, where ethics rounds were begun in 1979 and continue in the present. The essays in the first part of this volume place the ethical problems of treating mentally ill people in the context of the health care ethics movement and traditions of ethical decision making. The essays as a whole provide an explicit framework and guide to those wishing to institute clinical rounds centered on the ethical facets of patient care, and other forms of teaching about mental health ethics based on a case approach. We have written this volume with a view toward also helping those readers and teachers who do not have access to the type of clinical case material that can provide real-life examples from which to conduct ethical analyses.

We hope that the cases and essays adequately convey the gratification we feel as clinicians and teachers for the insight we have gained from the experiences of patients and therapists. Those experiences have helped us better appreciate the significance of ethical values in understanding and treating mental illness and in promoting mental health.

2

NEW PROBLEMS, NEW ETHICS: CHALLENGING THE VALUE STRUCTURE OF HEALTH CARE

IN THE MIDDLE of the 1960s, a revolution took place that pushed away the veil shrouding the ethical dilemmas of health care. It exposed not abuse, but misunderstanding, and a widespread unawareness of the ethical context of the relationships among medical personnel, patients, and society. Without some knowledge of this revolution in general medicine, the related developments in mental health cannot be fully understood.

HEALTH CARE AS A RIGHT

The ethics movement was the outcome of multiple events, linked by their focus on rights. Particularly important was the effort at the beginning of this century to equalize the quality of care among the diverse strata of American society.

A traditional attitude in the United States toward social provision of health care had been that meeting the basic needs of life was the responsibility of the individual. Society would intervene when an illness posed a long-term threat to a person's health, the care for the disease was time-consuming and placed substantial burdens on the family, or the disease posed a danger to the community. By these definitions, persons afflicted with tuberculosis, mental illness, and retardation were candidates for social support, and many hospitals were built during the 19th and 20th centuries to treat these disorders. Society also responded to the general medical needs of the poor by constructing institutions for their care: Indigency was a condition that legitimized social intervention.

The movement to give people broad access to health care, regardless of their specific illness or financial state, met with continued

3

resistance from the time it began in the early 20th century right up to 1960. Then, the rising cost of medical care dovetailed with a growing conviction that a particular segment of the population, the elderly, was particularly vulnerable to both illness and the large medical bills now accompanying it. The Democratic Party, with John F. Kennedy as its presidential nominee, caught wind of an emerging national consensus, which favored social assumption of the health care of the elderly, and supported a government-financed insurance scheme that would give this age group medical access and protection. This scheme was embodied in the 1965 Medicare Act. In the wave of social activism that was the hallmark of the Great Society, Medicaid legislation in 1966 consolidated the federal government's medical assistance plans for the poor.

Although the magnitude of this commitment of health service delivery by the federal government represented a policy departure, in essence, tradition was maintained. Once again, the country had opted to provide health care rights to well-defined groups having special needs and had rejected a policy giving broad health care coverage to all.

However, in the 1960s the fact that millions had acquired the right to health care resources through Medicare and Medicaid dramatically changed the government's view of its responsibility to oversee the nation's health. The government was no longer a bystander, but had become a responsible party with major obligations. For the first time in American history, "right to health care" was a familiar phrase in the political dialogue.

CIVIL RIGHTS FOR WOMEN AND ABORTION

Simultaneously with these events, a large civil rights movement, with significant origins in the 1950s, began to influence women's views of their position in society. In the early 1960s women began to ask, in an increasingly public and forceful manner, why the barriers to equal opportunity with men in all spheres of life should not be taken down.

A central question of interest to this movement was how women could approach their function as the bearer of children and yet retain a capacity for equal participation with men in the opportunities and rights of American society. This raised into the social consciousness of the 1960s the long-debated question of what the status of the fetus was and whose views – those of its mother, father, the state, or religion – should take precedence in deciding this question.

A strong argument was presented that a woman's central role in the process of fetal maturation and birth should make her the predominant figure in this decision. This debate generated one of the most prolonged, socially open, and productive discussions ever held on abortion. Difficult questions were raised concerning the meaning of personhood, the right of individuals to adjudicate decisions about their own biologic functions, and the right of the state to intervene in such matters.

Often the discussion was charged with great emotion. For those who believed the fetus was a person from the moment of conception, abortion represented killing. Others considered the viewpoints about the fetus to be so philosophically conflicting and bound in untestable religious tenet, that it seemed socially and morally desirable to give individuals relative freedom in deciding how to regard the fetus. This was the essential position taken by the U.S. Supreme Court in 1972 in *Roe v. Wade*. It permitted the woman and doctor to determine jointly whether abortion was reasonable during the first trimester of pregnancy. In the second trimester, the state was given the prerogative to protect the health of the mother. In the final trimester, the state might pass laws to protect the fetus.

By posing such questions in the 1960s, the debate on abortion led clinicians, among others, to analyze the meaning of personal rights, the definition and consequences of autonomy, and the boundaries of state power to intervene in decisions involving the body of the individual.

TECHNOLOGY AND ETHICS

Complementing these social movements in the 1960s was a technologic revolution in medicine, unparalleled in its breadth and complexity. This revolution affected attitudes toward three issues in particular: the allocation of resources, the definition of death, and the dilemma of justifying cessation of aggressive, life-sustaining therapy.

In 1944, Willem Kolff, a physician in Holland under Nazi occupation, used human beings to test a machine that cleansed the blood of toxic products accumulating as a result of kidney failure. The device was make-shift and intended only to assist the body's toxic waste disposal needs for a short period, during episodes of acute renal failure. It was ineffective in the first 14 patients tested. For the 15th patient, a woman, it proved to be a life-saving device.

By 1961 the machine was clinically perfected, with the addition of a shunt allowing the patient and machine to be connected for prolonged periods and filters to remove waste from the blood in a more effective way than in the past. Furthermore, drugs had been developed to prevent clotting when blood flowed through the system. Thus technically improved, the artificial kidney appeared at the Dialysis Center in Seattle, Washington. With thousands of people in the United States in the final stage of renal disease, the demand for therapy rapidly exceeded the supply of machines and the personnel to run them. The hospital staff was faced with the ethical problem of how to distribute a life-saving technological resource among desperate claimants, a type of situation Americans had not faced since World War II.

Those charged with making these choices decided to empanel an ethics committee composed of medical personnel and community representatives to develop guidelines for allocation, and to act on them. The rules they adopted to choose one person over another – particularly those aspects that weighed social merit and ability to pay – seemed unsatisfactory to social and medical critics. This committee labored mightily, under much stress, navigating in uncharted waters. Yet, in retrospect, it is clear that making choices of this sort using such guidelines is extremely difficult. Some critics began to urge that greater randomness be introduced into the process. Others called for a national program to support the financial needs of those in renal failure who were candidates for dialysis and transplantation. In 1972, such a program became law, eliminating the need to choose among patients having kidney disease. This legislation shifted the problem from the patient and ethics committee to society, which now contributes more than $2 billion in annual costs to support this program.

The artificial kidney was but one of a cohort of new technologies introduced into medicine in the 1960s that staved off death in the face of massive physiological collapse. These technologies included artificial respirators, monitoring machines, and more effective drugs, all of which gave medical staffs undreamed of power to keep the human body alive. These devices challenged the intellectual constructs medicine had fashioned to deal with death. To a physician or a nurse in the early 1960s death was simple and unequivocal – it was defined as the cessation of heart and lung functions and the absence of pupillary contraction in the presence of bright light. The tools used to diagnose this condition were simple – a stethoscope and a flashlight. However, once the technology was available to sustain these functions, such strategies and tools became obsolete. New concepts and other machines were needed. They emerged in 1966 in the notion of brain death and in the growing reliance on the electroencephalograph (EEG) to determine this condition. Death was now defined by criteria involving neurologic and brain function, partly viewed through the wave-form evidence of the EEG. The paradox of the heart and lungs working while the person who housed them was brain dead presented surreal images to medical staffs and families of the patients.

This new approach to death raised complex ethical questions concerning not only the definition of death itself, but also the nature of the medical heroics appropriate to life-threatening crises. In the past, the issue of whether to restrain therapy had been a subject of medical concern and debate. The ancient Greek dictum urging physicians "to help, or at least to do no harm," implied that the unrestrained use of medical force could lead to much suffering for the patient. Not harming, in this formulation, was as much a good as helping.

Although physicians and patients in previous ages grappled with this question, their engagements were sporadic and of short duration. The illness, usually unyielding to therapeutics if it was serious and acute, ended after a not too prolonged course. The therapeutics of the 1960s changed this pattern significantly. Strengthened by the advances of science, the new therapeutics, with the technology of rescue in its vanguard, fought off illness and staved off death. But at a high price. For those who did not begin to recover their normal functions within the space of weeks, each day increased the likelihood that the patient would not return to normal. If not recovery, if not death, what then? Lingering. Patients lingered in the twilight life of — *Better* vital function, continuing without hope or even consciousness. And *or worse off then dead?*

while they lingered, staff and family grew uneasy, perplexed, and embittered about the machines that at first were seen as agents of rescue.

This situation generated calls for reflection on the ethics of the matter and for action. Any action that would bring about some resolution seemed preferable to the waiting and the hopelessness that grew with it.

With the repeated occurrence of such events over a range of medical disasters, from accidents to cancer, many turned to the theory and practice of ethics for an approach that would reconfirm the validity of initially applying the new technological marvels to these disorders. It became clear that only a rational approach with an ethical basis for withdrawing therapy would deliver the relief to patients and families that medicine was expected to bring.

EXPERIMENTATION AND THE RIGHTS OF SUBJECTS

An event that dovetailed in the 1960s with the debate on therapeutics had to do with the science used to generate them. Experiments that used human subjects to test the effects of new therapies had taken place throughout medical history. What was new in this decade was the influence of experiments performed on humans by the Nazis in World War II, which drew attention to the dangers for the subjects in experimental investigations and to the obligations of scientists to guard against them. To this was added a growing sensitivity to ethical questions in medicine in general, which increased the scrutiny to which research on human subjects was subjected.

The outcome of the judicial deliberations concerning experimentation on human beings during World War II was the formulation of ten standards, known as the Nuremberg Code, that were to be observed in this activity. These standards were established in recognition of the need to inform subjects fully about the possible outcomes of their participation, and to make certain that investigators were morally obligated to ensure the subject's safety, independent of the consent process.

The standards helped investigators to clarify their obligations. But they were not by themselves adequate to prevent subjects from being harmed. In the late 1950s and 1960s, several widely publicized cases involving unethical practices in human studies led the U.S. Public Health Service to issue a regulation in 1966 requiring all hospitals and other medical institutions conducting research on human subjects to empanel committees of medical staff and laymen. Their purpose was twofold: to evaluate all human studies and ensure that they were designed so as to minimize harm to subjects; and to provide subjects with a full view of the possible dangers as well as benefit, so that their decision to enter a trial was "informed."

One of the cases that brought attention to the need for additional safeguards occurred in an institution for the mentally retarded called the Willowbrook State School. There, in the late 1950s, newly admitted children were fed hepatitis virus in an experiment designed to investigate the circumstances under which the disease occurred, evaluate the cogency of gamma globulin in reducing its occurrence, and test the induction of immunity by feeding hepatitis virus to gamma globulin-protected persons. The investigators justified the experiment on the basis of their experience that most of those entering the school got the infection, that it was a benign disease in children, that facilities were available at the school to provide good medical care in an isolation unit, that the experimentally induced disease would be milder than the natural infection (this turned out to be the case), and that consent for the study had been gained from parents of the subjects involved. Was such a proxy consent adequate? Should people such as children or the mentally retarded, who cannot give their own consent, be provided with additional procedural safeguards? What ethics should be guiding the research on such people (1)? The Willowbrook case stirred such questions.

Consent of the subject had been a central feature of the Nuremberg Code. However, since 1966 – when it was stipulated that all investigators must consider this issue before their research is approved – investigators have come to better understand and become more sensitive to their obligations to and the rights of subjects.

THERAPEUTIC ACTIVITIES AND THE RIGHTS OF PATIENTS

The focus on consent and the autonomy of the subject in experimentation stimulated investigators to explore these issues in relation

to the therapeutic activities of medicine. In the 1960s clinicians began
to examine how they treated the passage of information to patients.
In the 1970s there emerged a consensus that doctors had withheld
too much from patients in the past and that the patients had a right
to participate in important decisions affecting them.

This concern was reflected in a document published in 1973 by
the American Hospital Association, *Statement on a Patient's Bill of
Rights*. It emphasized the right of patients to have complete and clear
information concerning diagnosis, prognosis, and therapy. It called
on physicians to obtain the informed consent of patients before the
start of any therapy; that is, it asked them to stipulate the risks and
the expected length of incapacitation, and to let patients know about
the availability of significant alternative therapeutic options. Rights
to refuse treatment and to privacy and confidentiality were enum-
erated, along with information about bills and hospital rules. In
essence, the document represents an important and explicit public
statement concerning the enhanced role of patients in deciding the
terms of medical care.

THE ETHICS MOVEMENT IN MENTAL HEALTH

The ethics movement in health care also led those charged with
treating patients suspected of or having diminished capacity to evaluate the therapeutic alternatives, to review more critically than they
had in the past the terms under which they exercised paternalistic
oversight. Nowhere in health care was this more significant or difficult than in the field of mental health. Psychiatrists, social workers,
psychologists, and other mental health therapists began, as never
before, to question the ethical values under which they developed
relationships with patients, colleagues, society, and the state (2). A
number of issues were central to this discourse. One dealt with the
psychiatrist as "double-agent" (3). This issue in particular received
publicity in the early 1970s, as news reached the West of the use of
Soviet psychiatrists and psychiatry to quell political dissent by linking
it to mental illness and committing dissenters to mental hospitals as
patients. Other circumstances in which mental health therapists felt

divided loyalties and obligations – such as their work in the military, prisons, and schools – also received attention. Could they serve the needs of the institutions and the society they represented and still serve the needs of their soldier, prisoner, and student patients? And what about situations in which mental health therapists were asked by courts to evaluate or follow up on patients who had committed crimes? Should the privacy of a patient-therapist relationship be protected and reports on its content be withheld from interested and powerful parties? How could the therapist best serve the patient – by cooperating with authorities and giving them information, or by denying them access to it?

The problem of divided loyalty was also present in family therapy. To whom is the therapist responsible? How does the therapist treat confidentiality? Should children be protected by confidentiality in the same manner as adult members of the family? Therapists dealing with adolescents as single patients experienced the same problems and sought to clarify the ethical conflicts (4).

Conflicting loyalties also emerged with regard to involuntary commitment and treatment and the basic struggle in the field of mental health between autonomy and paternalism. Before the 1970s, the main criterion used to determine whether patients of no threat to others should be committed was the need for treatment, which was based upon a therapist's judgment of whether patients could care for themselves. During the 1970s, a shift occurred. The view of good, determined by the expert (therapist), was challenged by a view of good determined by the patient. In the dialogue about the possible harms of alternative modes of care, including confinement, the patient's voice received more attention than in the past. The rights of patients to assert what was in their interest, as they saw it, even if harm might occur to them, competed with the therapist's professed duty to prevent a harm deemed likely to occur if the treatment was opposed.

At the same time, patients who presented risks to others were creating even greater dilemmas for the therapists. Here, the need to protect society from the potentially harmful actions of a mentally ill patient clashed with the newly enhanced rights to autonomy of action and protection of the individual's freedoms. Like the issue of the double agent this raised the matter of whose welfare should concern the mental health therapist more – that of the patient or that of society and its members.

This dilemma arose in perhaps the most famous legal case involving psychiatry of this period – *Tarasoff* v. *Regents of the University of California*. On October 27, 1969, Prosenjit Poddar, a 25-year-old research assistant at the University of California, Berkeley, fatally stabbed Tatiana Tarasoff, a 20-year-old student, on the porch of her home. The parents of Tatiana brought a suit against the university regents, doctors, and campus police. They alleged that, two months earlier, the research assistant had confided his intention to kill Tatiana to a university psychologist. They alleged that at the psychologist's request, campus police had detained Poddar, but released him when he seemed rational. They also claimed that the psychologist's superior then requested that no further action be taken to detain Poddar, and nobody warned Tatiana of her peril.

On the first appeal of this case to the California Supreme Court, on December 23, 1974, the court ruled that a doctor has a legal duty to warn a potential victim such as Tatiana of a possible peril: "When a doctor or psychotherapist, in the exercise of his professional skill and knowledge, determines, or should determine, that a warning is essential to avert a danger arising from the medical or psychological condition of his patient, he incurs the legal obligation to give warning" (5).

The case was reheard by the California Supreme Court, which in its ruling given on July 1, 1976, enlarged the obligation of therapists, from a duty to *warn* to a duty to *protect*:

> When a therapist determines, or pursuant to the standards of his profession should determine, that his patient presents a serious danger of violence to another, he incurs an obligation to use reasonable care to protect the intended victim against such a danger. The discharge of this duty may require the therapist to take one or more of various steps depending upon the nature of the case. Thus it may call for him to warn the intended victim of the danger, to notify the police, or take whatever other steps are necessary under the circumstances. (6)

The decision thus argued that the public interest forced the value of confidential disclosure in patient-psychotherapeutic relations to yield to the value of avoiding danger to others. But a dissenting opinion in the case should be noted. Justice Clark argued that the decision would inhibit people from seeking psychiatric care and would harm the care given to those receiving therapy, for it restrained them from making the revelations required for effective therapy and thus damaged the bond of trust upon which therapeutic relationships are founded.

The mental health literature of the period also discussed the role of ethical values in basic decisions that institutions and therapists made about illness. Some works criticized the tradition in mental therapy of emphasizing the scientific advances of the field and of minimizing its ethical aspects. As Arieti noted: "Values always accompany and give special significance to facts and . . . when we deprive facts of their values, we fabricate artifacts which have no reality in human psychology" (7). Other works examined the values of the environment in which mental therapy was practiced. The values of the legal system were singled out as key variables affecting therapeutic decisions of the 1970s and 1980s, particularly in the dominance of the value of autonomy and freedom of the individual over the values of promoting health and giving compassion. Some therapists criticized this weighting. The doctrine of treating patients in the least restrictive environment and with the least intrusive intervention, Halleck wrote, "diminishes the possibility that the doctor can interact with the patient in the most useful manner" (8, p. 176). This balance of values affected not only the conduct of therapeutic relationships, but also the policy of therapeutic institutions:

> For over a decade now society has tended to deal with the problems of the deterioration of care in these institutions not by improving them but by devising a variety of legal methods for keeping people out of them. In following this direction, both liberal and conservative elements in society are able to convince themselves that they are not only furthering the value of freedom or individualism, but they are saving money as well!! (8, p. 179)

The values inherent in mental health theory and practice itself also stirred up discussion. Some argued, for example, that the value of contributing to the emotional growth of the patient inappropriately dominated the value of palliating symptoms or helping to sustain a marginal patient's existence.

There also appeared in the 1970s annotated versions of general codes of medical ethics as they applied to psychiatry. One of these was the American Psychiatric Association's first commentary on the Principles of Ethics of the American Medical Association (AMA), published in 1973. When a new AMA code appeared in 1980, it repeated the task. This latest commentary emphasized the need to avoid using relationships to gratify the emotional needs of the therapists; the difficulties in handling confidentiality; the questions raised in refusing to accept a patient; the need to inform a patient when the therapist's values interfered with the therapy; the problems of getting competent consent; the dilemmas of dealing with the media; the conflict and responsibilities as citizens in commenting, say, about the treatment of a public figure; and the need to maintain the patient's privacy (9). Similar annotations for psychiatrists were added to the Canadian Medical Association Code of Ethics (10). The disciplines of psychology (11), social work (12), and nursing (13) also developed detailed ethical codes.

For the therapeutic disciplines gathered under the umbrella of mental health, as for the rest of health care, the ethics movement stimulated providers and institutions to examine the role of values in determining actions. This has strengthened the ability of therapists to explore conflicting human needs, rights, and aspirations with their patients.

References

1. Ward, R., et al. (1958). Infectious hepatitis. *New England Journal of Medicine,* 258, 407–416.
2. Mills, D. H. (1984). Ethics education and adjudication within psychology. *American Psychologist,* 39(6), 669–675.
3. Steinfels, M. O., & Levine, C. (eds.). (1978, April). In the service of the state: The psychiatrist as double agent. A conference on conflicting loyalties cosponsored by the American Psychiatric Association and the Hastings Center/March 24–26, 1977. *Hastings Center Report Special Supplement.*
4. Miller, D. (1977). The ethics of practice in adolescent psychiatry. *American Journal of Psychiatry,* 134(4), 420–424.
5. Tarasoff v. Regents of the University of California, 529 P. 2d 553, 555 (Cal. 1974).

6. Tarasoff v. Regents of the University of California, 551 P. 2d 334, 340 (Cal. 1976).

7. Arieti, S. (1975). Psychiatric controversy: Man's ethical dimension. *American Journal of Psychiatry*, 132(1), 39–42.

8. Halleck, S. L. (1981). Covert values in the treatment of psychosis. *American Journal of Psychotherapy*, 35(2), 173–186.

9. American Psychiatric Association. (1981). *The principles of medical ethics with annotations especially applicable to psychiatry* (rev. ed.). Washington, D.C.

10. Mellor, C. (1980). The Canadian Medical Association code of ethics annotated for psychiatrists, the position paper of the Canadian Psychiatric Association. *Canadian Journal of Psychiatry*, 25, 432–438.

11. Ethical principles of psychologists. (1981). *American Psychologist*, 36(6), 633–638.

12. Code of Ethics – National Association of Social Workers. (1980). Approved by National Association of Social Workers (NASW), House Delegate Committee.

13. Code for nurses with interpretive statements. (1976). American Nurses Association, Publication G-56.

3

CONFLICT AND SYNTHESIS: THE COMPARATIVE ANATOMY OF ETHICAL AND CLINICAL DECISION MAKING

CLINICAL DECISION MAKING inevitably occurs not in discipline-specific isolation but in an ethical context. This chapter illustrates the ways in which the application of ethical principles, which represent the long-standing traditions of ethical decision making, may contribute to solving knotty problems in the clinical arena.

Although clinicians may not be aware of the specific philosophy they are espousing when they make a clinical decision, every clinical approach reflects some ethical position. That is, every treatment program embodies certain values, and each set of values is based on a model of what human beings are like and how, through their actions, they approach the dispensation of goodness. Each model uses a specific set of values and concepts in explaining how human choices have right-making and wrong-making consequences for their agents.

Conflict over which values should be promoted in treatment decisions is natural, as at times we all have conflicting internal values, and this conflict may be externalized into an interpersonal conflict between group members having otherwise common interests. But a conscious understanding of the ethical traditions that have influenced clinical decision making can help to enrich the clinical process and, in turn, its traditions can enrich and enlarge ethics. In mental health more than in any other area of medicine, as will be seen in our case example, the therapeutic alliance must avoid the Scylla of paternalism that can degenerate into coercion and the Charybdis of autonomy that can lead to abandonment. To do so, therapists must have an explicit understanding of clinical and ethical traditions and some knowledge of current legal standards, which together can serve to triangulate decision making under uncertainty (1–3).

To provide an overview of how ethical considerations influence

17

clinical decision making, we consult some of history's most illustrious ethicists. Beginning with a contemporary case, we call upon our consultants to offer guidance with the decision. (Of course, their "recommendations" are based on our extrapolations from their theoretical works.) Our selected group consists of Aristotle, John Stuart Mill, Immanuel Kant, G. W. F. Hegel, and G. E. Moore (3–6).

THE CASE

A 13-year-old girl who had been in psychotherapy for almost two years was presented at ethics rounds like those described in the following chapter. The presentation was being held because the therapist had completed training and consequently had to terminate with the patient. The patient, although referred to another therapist in the clinic, was reluctant to continue with anyone else.

The patient, A., had been living with her maternal grandmother, who, by all accounts, had made the child feel safe and loved. When A. was 6 years old, her father allegedly killed her mother one night "to save" the mother "from a worse fate." In the morning, he told A. that her mother was sleeping and took her out for a pleasant excursion.

A.'s father was convicted and spent the next seven years in jail. A. said she thought her father was innocent and had been framed. On a conscious level, she idealized her father. However, A. reported many nightmares about her father to her therapist. It appeared that on an unconscious level she realized that he was a man who had been convicted of murder and who might become dangerous again. A.'s father had visited with his daughter during brief leaves from jail. A. initially reported to her therapist many sexualized interactions with her father on these occasions. However, these sexualized interactions stopped almost two years ago.

A.'s father, who was being released from jail in two weeks, felt he deserved custody of his daughter and planned to apply to the court for custody. The patient stated that she wanted to live with her father. Furthermore, she asked the therapist to respect this decision by not revealing what she had reported concerning her father's earlier behavior toward her. A.'s grandmother was reluctant to oppose the father's wish for custody.

The therapist who presented the case identified two issues as problematic and offered them for discussion. First, she questioned whether she should act paternalistically, protect the patient and go against her expressed wishes, and tell the court what she had been told about the father's behavior, or whether she should respect the patient's wish for confidentiality and thus support her autonomy. In other words, how should the balance be struck between safety and freedom, between protection (paternalism) and autonomy (individualism)? As possible support for going against the patient's expressed wishes, the therapist wondered whether the the patient's fear of her father expressed in her dreams wasn't a better approximation of the patient's genuine feelings than her overt desire to live with him? Second, how could the therapist nourish the patient's true self by supporting the patient's growth and also ensure that the process could continue later *without* the therapist, as termination proceeded? This might be called the termination paradox: How can a process such as therapy, which depends on two people, one of whom is initially dependent on the other for growth, enable that person to become independent? Which of the patient's conflicting identifications (with the father, mother, or therapist) would provide an impetus to maturity and which would have to be surmounted to achieve this end? The therapist recognized that although these questions can be explored with the patient, such exploration cannot be guided solely by the clinical material, but necessarily involves a value-governed model of maturity. Depending on the patient's level of maturity and environment (especially her father and grandmother), the main focus of attention may be on conflicts related to survival, separation, self-assertion, and identity formation. How the patient resolves these conflicts – by predominantly using so-called more primitive or higher-level (e.g., self-assertion) defenses – itself reflects a hierarchy of values that is the product of the interaction between the nature of the individual and the supporting environment.

THE NATURALIST POSITION

Aristotle (384–322 B.C.). Aristotle espoused a naturalist morality; that is to say, he believed human beings can achieve virtue and happiness by fulfilling their natural capacities. His treatises on ethics rapidly gained currency during his lifetime and continue to be influential today. Aristotle wished to develop basic principles of human conduct. Aristotle believed that "the good" is happiness, an activity of the soul. The good of persons, their happiness, is tied in with the *function* particular to them. Human beings are unique by virtue of their reason: The good person is led by reason, a uniquely human trait. The use of reason in ethical dilemmas cannot, however, help us resolve them conclusively and with certainty. What is reasonable is learned through observation and experience and is achieved by identifying the *mean* between extremes. A person has a distinctive function to fulfill or end to achieve, and every action aims at some good. All of us have within ourselves the principles of good. These principles can be discovered by study and attained through behavior. People who are good are those who fulfill their function. Discovering what is good is linked to discovering the unique functions of one's human nature. Thus morality involves habits, right choice, and correct behavior.

The matter of choice is most relevant. People are capable of two types of reasoning, theoretical and practical: Without these, we would have no moral capacity. Although we all have a natural capacity for right behavior, we can only reach this potential through knowledge, a kind of thought that culminates in an act or a choice.

Applying Aristotle in this case, the therapist must determine, through reason and contemplation, what her job or function is with regard to the patient. She must call upon skills of observation and her experiences as a therapist in order to make a good choice. The crucial question is *What is her function as a therapist?* Is it to encourage autonomy in her patient or to protect her? The therapist has the moral capacity to make the right choice by studying the theoretical issues and practical concerns. Since each of the moral virtues – one of which is justice (and a just choice) – is a rationally determined mean between excess and deficiency, determining the *mean* between freedom and safety requires careful consideration of all the relevant facts in a given situation.

In this context, Aristotle's recommendation might well be to avoid embracing either extreme: granting the patient absolute autonomy or aggressively intervening in a paternalistic manner. Thus, while respecting the patient's desire for confidentiality, the therapist might encourage a more appropriate caretaker to seek custody of the child. As the pioneer 20th-century child psychoanalyst, Anna Freud, wrote, that choice should be determined by "who, among *presently available* adults, is or has the capacity to become a psychological parent and thus will enable the child to feel wanted. We can predict that the adult most likely suited for the role is the one, if there be one, with whom the child had and continues to have an affectionate bond rather than one of otherwise equal potential who is not yet in a primary relationship with the child" (8).

In this case the provider might well be the child's maternal grandmother, if only she could be supported in disentangling the love she had for her murdered daughter from the hatred she had for the offspring of her daughter's murderer. In any custody battle she will need to be supported to be at her best, so as to work through her own conflicting feelings and identifications. She and the child have had a relationship of affection. Although outwardly indifferent as to custody, she is in a better position to help the child continue to feel wanted than the father, who wants the child because he feels he "deserves" custody. This not only represents a satisfactory compromise between autonomy and independence in the immediate situation, but promises to generate a similar equilibrium through the child's formative years.

THE NOTION OF DUTIES AND OBLIGATIONS

Immanuel Kant (1724–1804). Moral worth exists when a person acts from a sense of duty: Yet, it is not enough that an act should be one that "duty" or obligation mandates. Every individual knows which choice is morally right, yet each of us struggles with right action in the face of temptation. The essential conflict lies between scientific explanations of natural events and our sense of moral responsibility for our actions. Kant's philosophy is an attempt to reconcile the mechanistic causal interpretation of events with freedom in human behavior. Nothing is intrinsically good except a good will. The moral intentions of an individual are more important than what the individual actually does. What makes an act morally good is the willingness of the person to perform the act. Rational people try to do what they ought to do out of a duty to moral law, but morality is clearly impossible without freedom of will or choice.

In the case of A., Kant might identify a duty to act toward others as we would have others act toward us, captured by the question, "Do we want to be protected (dependent) or to be allowed to act autonomously (independent)?" Both states exist in people; in fact, A.'s dreams bring up the conflict between autonomy and the wish for protection (here Kant would agree with Anna Freud's father, Sigmund Freud) (9). There exists, in people, a conflict between passion (id) and reason (ego) (9). The therapist, as well as the patient, experiences such conflicts. The therapist can help A. (and herself) to become a free moral agent by exploring with her and helping her attempt to reconcile hitherto unconscious passions and ideals. In bringing them to consciousness, the therapist helps her bear the pain of mourning what cannot be reconciled, thereby mediating passion with reason.

Kant would perhaps argue that a therapist's duty is to help the patient explore the issues and that to intervene against the patient's wishes is to depart from that duty. After all this would be what the therapist herself, in the patient's situation, would most likely want. It is also the course of action most likely to promote rational decision making on the part of the patient.

TRUTH AND RATIONALITY

G. W. F. Hegel (1770–1831). For Hegel, reality is a synthesis of all truths, achieved through the consciousness of a dialectic in which we move from an initial position to its opposite, and ultimately to a position that encompasses both. The dialectic, a process by which the synthesis of opposites can proceed, consists of the thesis, the antithesis, and the synthesis. The thesis represents one concept, the antithesis opposes it, and the synthesis resolves the conflict between the thesis and antithesis. The synthesis resolves the conflict by keeping what is truthful and valuable in both. In all, this makes for a triadic dialectic. Truth and goodness are not static, but ever changing throughout the history of dialectic development.

In terms of ethics, morality consists of acting in concordance with the moral principles embodied in the spirit of one's age, that is, in concordance with what is most highly developed in one's own society and institutions; ethics is really social ethics. Greater than the need for individual autonomy is the need to be part of a social whole. Substantial freedom consists in the identification of personal ideals with the best ideals of one's state.

As for the case of A., the dialectic method – which is based on insight and interpretation, more than empiricism – offers an approach to a decision. Consider the following structure:

Thesis: The patient wants to make autonomous decisions – she wishes to be able to protect herself – and this leads her to an unconscious identification with her father as protector, and thus, her conscious wish to live with her father. This comes to be expressed at termination, when she feels helpless and is filled with rage as she experiences the therapist as abandoning her. In the face of such helplessness, she wishes to turn the tables and render the abandoning therapist helpless. Her identification is now with her father as aggressor.

Antithesis: The patient wishes to be dependent and protected – to seek help from the therapist. The nightmares signify fear and telling the therapist about her father's sexualized interactions with her indicates her desire for protection, as she identifies with her father's previous victim – her mother. At termination the patient reexperiences her own childlike state of helplessness at the time of the murder.

Synthesis: The patient should be helped to get the best support from identifications with both father and mother. After termination, the patient will retain her identification with how the therapist responds to the dilemma confronting her. Thus the therapist's response must steer a course between omnipotent interventionism and helpless neutrality, while acknowledging the social context of the decision. The therapist might say: "Your safety comes first. At the same time I respect your wish for autonomy. Given what *you* told me, I believe that you are not aware that what is right for you is to live with your grandmother. Perhaps we can find some room for negotiation. Sooner or later you will come to realize that this solution will enable your true self to come into being." By giving such a view, Hegel would be emphasizing what modern object relations therapists such as Winnicot have called the importance of the therapist providing the patient with a "holding environment," in which the patient's ability to synthesize internal conflict can grow even as it is negotiated interpersonally (10).

This synthesis would require the therapist's active intervention in court.

THE UTILITARIAN POSITION

John Stuart Mill (1808–1873). Mill, building on the work of Jeremy Bentham and John Locke, took the classic utilitarian position: The "greatest happiness is the greatest good." One course of action is better than another if it results in a greater balance of pleasure over pain and worse if the opposite is its consequence. Acts are right if they produce good consequences and wrong if they produce bad ones: One assesses the net of good consequences minus bad ones for each person to determine the total net good. One must take into account the certainty of benefits and harms as well as their duration, seeking the greatest good for the greatest number. This is the essence of utilitarianism or consequentialism.

Utility emphasizes the interests of each individual in harmony with the interests of all, the quantity and the quality of pleasures, and the good of the whole. Happiness is the ultimate goal, and we ought to choose – that is, it is our moral duty to pursue – those acts that produce the most good (an act is good or right according to how much happiness it produces). What offers proof that an end is desirable is that people strive for it.

In our case, Mill might weigh the consequences of choosing actively to intervene or not, and also the consequences of A. living with her father versus A. living apart from him and with her grandmother. This approach would enable one to make the choices that would yield the greater balance of pleasure over pain for the greatest number of people. The degree of certainty regarding benefits and harm, their magnitude, and their duration would influence the trade-off. In more modern terms, a technique called decision analysis has attempted to quantify these terms as an aid to reaching optimal decisions (11).

Consider the following:

A. wishes to live with her father. Her father wishes to live with A. (This is certain).

A. does not want to live with her grandmother. Her grandmother does not particularly care to have A. live with her. (This is certain.)

A. might be in danger living with her father. (This is uncertain.)

A.'s growth would be facilitated by being allowed to make the choice. (This is certain.)

A. would incur internal, psychological damage for the rest of her life by having to give up the part of herself that identifies with her father. (This is almost certain.)

Whether the net good favors allowing her to make the choice and live with her father or intervening to prevent this depends on the relative importance assigned to the competing values of freedom and safety. Relying on such a calculation might embolden Mill to recommend, if negotiations fail, letting the patient live with her father (12).

THE INTUITIONIST POSITION — THE NOTION OF THE GOOD

G. E. Moore (1873–1958). Addressing such questions as "What kinds of actions ought we to perform?" and "What kinds of things ought to exist for their own sake?" Moore proposed that intrinsically good things ought to exist for their own sake. Even given the impossibility of defining "good," a person has the contemplative ability to recognize what is intrinsically good. Although nothing can prove intrinsic goodness, its existence can be made apparent: That is, although intrinsic goodness is indefinable, you know it when you are faced with it. In terms of the question, "What kinds of actions ought we to perform?" empirical proof or disproof is needed to determine the answer. This position may seem mechanistic, in that it denies conflict and presumes that right answers are identifiable; yet Moore appears to hold that a course of action is right if it both causes the "most good" *and* yields consequences that are intrinsically good.

Consequently, for this case, Moore might ask, "Which is the best action?" This question poses a dilemma, since preventing murder and enhancing growth are both intrinsically good. The crux is, which action causes the most good, given the intrinsic goodness of both. When both choices are intrinsically good, the correct approach must be intuited, largely from evaluating the consequences. If we were to insist that Professor Moore leave us with a final recommendation, he might say: "I must remind you that families are by no means always the benign entities that some would claim. In your own age, R. D. Laing has argued that the price for a united family may be the death of the individual (13). Common sense tells us that where there is life, happiness is possible, but where there is no life, there can be no happiness. Thus let us ensure the patient's physical safety first, and if this produces, as an unavoidable by-product, emotional injury to either the patient or the other parties, we can deal with that in turn."

ETHICAL VERSUS LEGAL DECISION MAKING

A hidden element of our case – less hidden than it would have been in previous decades – is that practitioners face the threat of liability for a bad outcome following their deliberations. Today the careful weighing of ethical issues is not uncommonly concluded with the query, "Yes, but what does the law prescribe, allow, or prohibit?" And so in this case discussion, the temptation is to look to the law for guidance in determining the best decision. However, such a "flight to law" does not obliterate the ethical and clinical issues the case raises (14).

The goal of legal decision making is the dispensation of justice. The outcome or resolution of legal disputes is far from predictable and certain, but rather a matter of probability. One reason for this uncertainty is doubt about the facts – how they are revealed, the veracity of their revelation, and how they are construed by the decision makers. A second reason for uncertainty lies in the nature of the law itself. The legal rules are pliable, so that whether a particular rule applies to a particular case is a matter of interpretation and judgment.

The law and the legal system stand as attempts to shape ideal standards of conduct and (indirectly) morality for modern society. The law serves as interpreter of the ethical concepts of morality and justice. Legal decision making of the Anglo-American variety attempts to resolve conflict by an adversarial system. Each party to the dispute presents facts and seeks to show how they fit the rules derived from legislation, precedent, or public policy that will favor its desired outcome. Empirically testing hypotheses to arrive at truth is not commonly a part of legal reasoning. At the same time, critical legal decision making in its concern for precedent, the finding of fact, and hypothetical cases is not immune from considerations such as prior probabilities, simplicity, data gathering, and "gedank" experiments that characterize scientific and clinical discourse (15–16).

The interrelationship between the legal, clinical, and ethical discourses can be seen in the manner in which the law articulates standards for negligence in determining professional malpractice. For professional groups, the law has to do with standards of professional care: Two possibilities are the community standard and the reasonable practitioner standard. The latter emphasizes not only what kind of care most practitioners *do* provide, as does the former, but also what kind of care practitioners *ought* to provide, given what science has to offer. When this question is asked not only in the light of science, which gives us a sense of the probabilities, but also in the light of our values, then we have a third possibility, the risk–benefit approach to standards of care. This last legal standard, often called the "Learned Hand Rule," resembles the ethical position characterized by John Stuart Mill's utilitarianism.

These touchstones are used by law to establish what constitutes the "correct actions" in a given clinical situation, from one point of view. That is to say, this is how the law endorses ethical positions. But the critical point here is that the ethical approach to reasoning is no more reducible to the legal one than it is to the purely scientific or clinical.

ETHICAL DECISION MAKING AND THE PROBLEM OF UNCERTAINTY: THE TWO PARADIGMS

If ethics is to provide not merely a theoretical guide but also a practical guide to right actions, an additional factor must be considered: the inherent uncertainty of clinical practice. To address this question, one must first consider the two major models of reasoning involved in clinical decision making and their widely divergent approaches to dealing with uncertainty.

Although some clinicians consider clinical work to be akin to science, others argue that it is both more and less than a science: more, because the experience of illness involves human feelings and life; and less, because science is exact and predictable and mental health care (and the broader area of medical care in general) is not.

Despite this definitional dilemma, researchers in the area of clinical decision making have borrowed from science, particularly from 20th-century physics, a new way of approaching clinical care – they view it as a science of probability rather than a science of certainty (17). Even the field of physics, where Newton's laws once provided the framework for our knowledge of precise causes and effects and where prediction was thought to be possible with certainty, is no longer considered a mechanistic science of certainty, but an uncertain science of probability (see Table 1). What is important is not just the name or definition, but the fundamental assumptions that this shift from such a mechanistic to a probabilistic paradigm signifies.

A "paradigmatic shift," or change in the fundamental assumptions and procedures of science, usually occurs when the older paradigm can no longer reliably solve the problems at hand. Mental health care, along with physics, has changed tremendously in this century. The science of mental health care has been transformed by revolutionary technology, which has created the expectation that previously intractable disorders of character or psychobiology can be treated in the hope of not only relieving suffering, but even of finding a cure. With rising hopes has come disappointment and its fruits – mental health practitioners have been hard hit by malpractice suits. In reaction there has been increasingly widespread use of defensive, nontherapeutic practices. Clinicians have had to abandon their wishes for certainty in regard to clinical decision making – for the new technology has paradoxically made outcomes more hopeful but less certain. The expectations of patients and their families for perfectly predictable results as the end-product of the new technology have come to be as formidable an obstacle to a therapeutic alliance as the implacable hopelessness that can accompany chronic illness.

Therapists have tried to improve upon their decision-making rationales of the past and employ the newer probabilistic paradigm that accepts a degree of uncertainty as part of reality. Yet, in the case discussion we restricted our consultants' opinions to approaches that assumed that key factors could be defined with certainty. This belies the real world. The practical results of applying our consultants'

Table 1. *Mechanistic and probabilistic paradigms*

<hr>

Mechanistic

1. *Deterministic causation*
   Requires that for each observed effect, the scientist try to isolate one cause or many causes to explain the effect.
   Assumes the list of causes to be complete and the combination of causes static.
   Presupposes a static, one-person system.

2. *Experimentum crucis*
   Looks for one test that definitively establishes the deterministic causal relationship.
   Assumes that cause-and-effect relationships are 100 percent predictable and exact; and that there is no distortion by the observer.

3. *Objective-subjective dichotomy*
   Accepts only objective knowledge as reliable.
   Assumes objective knowledge to be independent of the observer.

Probabilistic

1. *Probabilistic causation*
   Recognizes that causes may interact differently at different times; thus the identical effects may have different causes.
   Acknowledges that causes operate to some degree by chance.
   Accepts uncertainty as inherent in causal relationships.
   Presupposes a dynamic two-person system.
   Understands that one of the sources of uncertainty is that to study a process is to intervene in it; thus the uncertainty is heightened.

2. *Experimentation as principled gambling*
   Holds that if patterns of cause and effect are subject to chance and change, no one experiment is "crucial."
   Endorses action based on hypotheses that appear to be true, good, and justified according to assigned probabilities and values.

3. *Continuity of the objective and subjective probabilistic causation*
   Admits that there is a subjective component to objective data and vice versa.

<hr>

ethical theories change drastically once the irreducibility of clinical uncertainty is acknowledged. We must abandon the wish for an omniscient consultant figure who can tell us the right thing to do and then omnipotently guarantee that tragic outcomes will be avoided if we follow his advice (18). As we begin to tolerate uncertainty, we come to recognize that we cannot be sure of avoiding regret or self-criticism for having chosen actions that seem ethically repugnant from the vantage point of the certainty of hindsight. In this context we can see that certainty is not possible either for the clinician (who is concerned about what choice will best protect the patient's growth) or for the patient (who is concerned about what choice will best enhance her growing autonomy). The most that our consultants have to offer are languages for exploring ethical conflict. The most that our clinical science has to offer is a framework for integrating that discussion into clinical practice. Neither *dictates* that one or another choice will be seen as virtuous in hindsight by others, or even by oneself. But if this is all, then it is quite a lot more than admitted by those who assert that if uncertainty exists, then "anything goes," relativism reigns supreme, and ethical and clinical theories are irrelevant to clinical practice.

On the contrary, in what follows we shall see that integrating ethical positions into a probabilistic framework enriches both the dialogue *between* parties – be it the alliance model of the clinical process or the adversary model of the legal process – and the *internal* dialogue by which the therapist and patient each comes to maturity by acknowledging to oneself, "This is what I can live with." In doing so, we can still use ethical theories, criteria for scientific reasoning, and legal precedent to fix our *initial* positions. We can use the experience embodied in these traditions to remind us of lacunae in our dialogue and to persuade us to change a clinical course if we find ourselves sailing into waters others have found treacherous. But the shoals of reality are sufficiently shifting that our navigational charts are an aid rather than a substitute for keeping a careful lookout. Moreover, we must modify our charts as we continue our voyage. We now explore how our chart of the course to be taken in this case needs to be further modified to take into account the clinical irreducibility of uncertainty.

Let us analyze our ethics case using the two models of decision

Table 2A. *Case example analyzed using the mechanistic model*

Criterion 1

Deterministic causation

The patient's inability to acknowledge that her father killed her mother and his current threat to her is the basic cause of the patient's neurosis and the current ethical conflict.

Criterion 2

Experimentum crucis

The patient's failure to acknowledge openly the potential threat posed by her father confirms that it is one of the main sources of her problems. This behavior demonstrates conclusively her inability to make reasonable decisions for herself and the need for the therapist to make those decisions for her.

Criterion 3

Objective-subjective dichotomy

The patient's spoken desires reflect her true wishes and indicate she is capable of recognizing reality; her dreams are irrelevant to these functions.

making, albeit with inevitable oversimplification. We begin with the mechanistic model in Table 2A.

The trouble with the mechanistic approach is that it reduces clinical reality and ethical conflict to a fruitless search for a "quick fix." That fix can take the shape of finding the answer in "natural law," whether that law happens to be a simplified version of clinical or ethical theory, or legal doctrine. In whatever ethical language the choice is framed, the discussion comes to be about abstract, isolated entities rather than about therapists and patients in relationships. These abstract entities come to be even further removed from the relationships when persons are considered, or consider themselves as having a certainty of will or interest that, from what we know of the nature of mind in society, is a mere fiction. Mental health involves first the capacity to engage in a dialogue with oneself as well as others when there is a disharmony between one's wishes and what can reasonably be said to be in one's best interest, and second the capacity to change. Clinicians who turn to ethics seeking to be "scientific" about their choices tend to reduce the possibility of dialogue and of change. Ethicists, such as "rights theorists," who speak of fictitious people who have only "the right to choose or to will" or the "right to protection of interests" forget that real people may have conflicting wishes and rights. In our case, the conflict is between the patient's wish to be with her father and her wish to grow safely. To say that the clinician who pays heed only to the former is being respectful of the patient's autonomy is to pay lip service to the concept of the patient's autonomy while disassociating the patient into a fictitious, conflict-free entity for the sake of our own peace of mind. To say that the therapist is being protective when she asks only how the patient can best be protected is to ignore the reality that the patient must ultimately learn to protect herself and requires support in making her own decision to do so. The clinician who implicitly adopts an oversimplified ethical position together with a mechanistic paradigm of clinical science is in danger of iatrogenically exacerbating the situation, and of foreclosing the possibility that the patient may learn to synthesize internally conflicting wishes via external negotiation.

Consider now the probabilistic approach, as presented in Table 2B.

THE INTERACTION OF ETHICS AND CLINICAL SCIENCE

How do the ethical and clinical approaches relate, and how is their relationship affected by the model of decision making chosen? In order to answer these questions we return to the ethical positions of our consultants. Their ethical positions do not translate directly into clinical decisions. Rather, their recommendations about the key *questions* that must guide clinical decision making come to be relevant only when integrated with the model of decision making employed in clinical practice.

Table 3 illustrates the interactions between the clinical and ethical approaches to decision making and justification. The choice of key questions has more to do with the basic values one wishes to justify

Table 2B. *Case example analyzed using the probabilistic model*

Criterion 1

Probabilistic causation

The patient's difficulties may stem from several sources. She may sense the danger from her father, but also from her grandmother's wish to abandon her, and may experience termination with the therapist as yet another abandonment, on a par with her mother's death. The external danger of being unprotected and the internal danger of losing part of herself (her identification with her father) must both be considered. The process of growth of a gender identity through adolescence involves an identification with the mother as victim.

Criterion 2

Experimentation as principled gambling

The father's role in the etiology of the patient's problems cannot be demonstrated by any single set of behaviors, but must be inferred from the totality of the circumstances. Since together these suggest that other factors also play some role, it cannot be assumed that the patient is incapable of making her own decisions simply because she fails to acknowledge the threat represented by her father. Therapy can only proceed if the therapist is open to the patient's associations and is guided by them in selecting the possible causative factors to examine, on the chance that they may play a role in the patient's difficulties. Exploring and mastering this process must be done *with* rather than *to* the patient. Thoughts, wishes, and fantasies will enable the patient to exercise increasing amounts of responsibility in making her own decisions. *Both* the therapist and the patient will be transformed to some degree by the process of observation, exploration, and dialogue.

Criterion 3

Continuity of objective and subjective probabilistic causation

By concentrating on one set of data, the objective – what the father did and what the patient says – we devalue the equally important subjective data with regard to what we can feel with the patient and what the patient wishes, albeit conflictually. Conversely, the subjective road is no sure way to the truth. What comes up in sessions with the therapist is no more reflective of the truth than the wishes disguised in the patient's dreams, and vice versa.

Table 3. *Interactions of ethics and clinical science*

Ethics	Clinical science (key questions)
Aristotle, naturalist	*Mechanistic paradigm*: How can one be the value-free clinician in search of the mean?
	Probabilistic paradigm: How can clinicians become conscious of their values and of the role they play in helping patients define and reach the desired mean?
Kant, notion of duties and obligations	*Mechanistic paradigm*: What is a clinician's duty to a patient?
	Probabilistic paradigm: What are the clinician's duties to a patient and what are the patient's duties to herself? What choice should a clinician make when there are conflicting duties and thus uncertainty?
Hegel, notion of natural rights	*Mechanistic paradigm*: What is the patient's natural right? (The answer to this question dictates the right clinical choice.)
	Probabilistic paradigm: When, as is inevitable, a person's rights conflict, e.g. when self-protection is in conflict with autonomy, how can the person be helped to work through the conflict maturely?
Mill, utilitarian	*Mechanistic paradigm*: What techniques, e.g., decision analysis, can be used as the experimentum crucis to learn what the best decision is?
	Probabilistic paradigm: How can any technique, e.g., decision analysis, be a basis for ongoing dialogue and experimentation rather than a fixed decision?
Moore, intuitionist notion of good	*Mechanistic paradigm*: How can one intuitively determine with certainty the good action of a therapist or of a patient?
	Probabilistic paradigm: Since what is good is by no means certain, how can it be continually reevaluated between therapist and patient?

than with a particular clinical method. Ethical arguments, regardless of the choice of terms (be it risks and benefits, duties and obligations, or rights and interests) ultimately rest on the wish to advance basic values. However, an ethical approach (or a combination of approaches) does not, particularly under the probabilistic model, provide *the* answer to the clinician's dilemma of how to act. Rather, it frames the inquiry that the clinician will undertake with the patient, although in doing so it may also implicitly define the universe of options.

The major barriers to reasonable use of ethical principles in clinical practice are (1) ambivalent, unrecognized value conflict within oneself (patient or therapist), and (2) an overriding desire for certainty. Unrecognized conflict prevents one from asking the key questions, leaving decision making to be a process driven by impulse. In that context, the concept of the unconscious is particularly relevant to clinical work and is critical to an understanding of ethics. We stated earlier that conscious understanding of ethical positions and traditions will help us to make better-informed decisions or choices; in much the same way, exploration of the unconscious and awareness of individual values, ideals, passions, and wishes may help individuals reach wiser personal decisions. The desire for certainty, an illusory and unattainable goal, can be mastered through a similar exploration of the limits and opportunities inherent in existence (18–21).

Psychotherapy seeks to give people the capacity to bear uncertainty and conflict through the therapeutic alliance; thus, both therapist and patient must mourn their wishes for certainty. The therapeutic alliance encourages dialogue and ultimately expands the internal arena where intrapsychic dialogue can take place. The hidden self, through this process, becomes conscious; the true self emerges on the social stage.

THE CLINICAL RELATIONSHIP AS AN ETHICAL POSITION

The framework within which clinical decision making occurs is the therapist-patient relationship. Here is where ethical principles and clinical desiderata are joined to reach treatment decisions. Yet, notice that the therapist-patient relationship itself is not formed in a value-neutral way. To the extent that the relationship is structured to

Table 4. *Effects of three approaches to the therapeutic relationship*

Clinical-ethical position	Dogmatic paternalism	Automatic autonomy	Tolerance of conflict and uncertainty
Therapeutic stance	Therapeutic reliance	Therapeutic abandonment	Therapeutic alliance
Relationship model	"Father knows best"	"Patient knows best"; "consumer choice"; laissez-faire	Shared uncertainty
Consequences for ethics	Social sovereignty	Sovereignty of the self	Encourages integration of traditional ethical principles into individual decision making
Consequences for relationship	Precludes empathy Fosters dependence Prevents autonomy	Engenders oppositionality Fosters counterdependence Leads to pseudoautonomy	Empathy Fosters interdependence Enhances autonomy

Affective consequences	Induces patient regression Interferes with dialogue Disappointment	Induces patient rejection Interferes with dialogue Frustration	Induces growth Encourages dialogue Acceptance of finitude, involving mourning and joy
Legal consequences	Unwarranted malpractice suits Defensive medicine: over-testing and increased patient risk; therapist's identification with the legal system (e.g., defensive use of informed consent)		Malpractice suits limited to actual negligence Best clinical judgment in selective use of procedures for patient's benefit
Outcome of therapy	One adult: the therapist	One adult: the patient	Two adults: therapist and patient

support one or another ethical value, the outcome of the decision-making process may be all but preordained.

Decision making depends a great deal on one's position with respect to and relationship with the other person in a dyad (22–23). We have all had the experience of making difficult choices. At times, we yearn for a substitute parent (doctor, lawyer, therapist) to make us feel safe and protected, someone we can trust to make a choice for us. However, both therapeutic reliance and its antithesis, therapeutic abandonment, are very different from allowing a patient to work in a personal therapeutic relationship or alliance. Table 4 illustrates these points.

The preceding chapter noted the social concordance between the evolution of the concern with ethical conflicts in medicine and the conflicts around confidentiality encountered in the treatment of adolescents. This chapter serves as an illustration of the point so eloquently emphasized by Erik Erikson that individual–family conflicts around individuation and identity formation during adolescence mirror and are mirrored by individual–institutional conflicts (24, 25). The next chapter offers a practical guide for institutional efforts in education for growth in the midst of ethical conflict and uncertainty.

The rigid adherence to either a uniformly paternalistic position or one that mindlessly encourages autonomy forces decision making into a straitjacket. Other values and ethical principles must bow to these preeminent values; conflict is not tolerated. But an ongoing relationship that accepts uncertainty provides a forum in which ethical concerns can be given proper consideration (1).

Law recognizes uncertainty in a person's relationship with other people; medical science recognizes uncertainty in a person's relationship with nature; clinical work recognizes uncertainty in a person's relationship with him- or herself. Decision making – be it clinical, intrapsychic, or legal – is directly influenced by the ethical positions and traditions that we hold and know. These traditions have enriched decision making in clinical practice and law. In turn their practical application in these broad disciplines can enrich the field of ethics. The importance of coming to know ethics, then, is that it enables us to discover and critique value positions and conflicts; ethics teaches us the questions to ask in exploring these influences on our decision-making behavior. An understanding of ethics allows us to be more conscious of and to bear the responsibility for what we choose and what we choose to leave behind. Thus we can come to know ourselves, even if such knowledge resembles that of Hegel's "owl of Minerva," which "flies only at dusk."

References

1. Bursztajn, H., Feinbloom, R. I., Hamm, R. M., & Brodsky, A. (1981). *Medical choices, medical chances – how patients, families and physicians can cope with uncertainty.* New York: Delacourt/Seymour Lawrence.
2. Katz, J. (1984). *The silent world of doctor and patient.* New York: The Free Press.
3. Stone, A. A. (1984). *Law, psychiatry and morality: Essays and analysis.* Washington, D.C.: American Psychiatric Press.
4. Bronstein, D. J., Krikorian, Y. H., & Wiener, P. P. (Eds.). (1972). *Basic problems in philosophy.* Englewood Cliffs, N.J.: Prentice-Hall.
5. Lavine, T. Z. (1984). *From Socrates to Sartre: The philosophic quest.* New York: Bantam Books.
6. MacIntyre, A. (1966). *A short history of ethics.* New York: Macmillan.
7. Stumpf, S. E. (1975). *Socrates to Sartre. A history of philosophy.* New York: McGraw-Hill.
8. Goldstein, J., Freud, A., & Solnit, A. J. (1973). *Beyond the best interest of the child.* New York: Free Press.
9. Freud, S. (1926). Inhibitions, symptoms, and anxiety. Reprinted in *The complete psychological works of Sigmund Freud,* standard edition, vol. 20, pp. 77–177. London: Hogarth Press, 1957.
10. Winnicott, D. W. (1965). *The maturational process and the facilitating environment.* New York: International Universities Press.
11. Raiffa, H. (1968). Decision analysis: Introductory lectures on choices under uncertainty. Reading, Mass.: Addison-Wesley.
12. Szasz, T. (1960). The myth of mental illness. *American Psychologist, 15*:113–118.
13. Laing, R. D., & Cooper, D. G. (1964). *Sanity, madness and the family: Vol. 1. Families of schizophrenics.* London: Tavistock.
14. Gutheil, T. G. (1979). Legal defense as ego defense: A special form of resistance in the therapeutic process. *Psychiatric Q, 51*:251–256.
15. Frank, J. (1970). *Law and the modern mind.* (6th ed.). Gloucester, Mass.: Peter Smith.
16. Dworkin, R. (1977). *Taking rights seriously.* Cambridge, Mass.: Harvard University Press.
17. Bursztajn, H., & Hamm, R. M. (1979). Medical maxims – two views of science. *Yale Journal of Biological Medicine, 52*:483–486.
18. Gutheil, T. G., Bursztajn, H., & Brodsky, A. (1984). Malpractice prevention through the sharing of uncertainty: Informed consent and the therapeutic alliance. *New England Journal of Medicine, 311,* 49–51.
19. Rako, S., & Mazer, H. (Eds.). (1980). *Semrad: The heart of a therapist.* New York: Jason Aronson.

40   *H. J. Bursztajn, T. G. Gutheil, and B. Cummins*

20. Modell, A. H. (1984). *Psychoanalysis in a New Context*. New York: International Universities Press.
21. Freud, S. (1916). On Transience. Reprinted in *The complete psychological works of Sigmund Freud*, standard edition, vol. 14, pp. 305–307. London: Hogarth Press, 1957.
22. Bursztajn, H., Hamm, R. M., Gutheil, T. G., & Brodsky, A. (1984). The decision-analytic approach to medical malpractice law. *Medical Decision Making*, 4:401–414.
23. Hamm, R. M., Clark, J. A., & Bursztajn, H. (1984). Psychiatrists' thorny judgements. *Medical Decision Making*, 4:425–447.
24. Erikson, E. (1963). *Childhood and society*, 2nd edition. New York: Norton.
25. Erikson, E. (1962). *Youngman Luther: A study in psychoanalysis and history*. New York: Norton.

4

SOLVING CLINICAL PUZZLES: STRATEGIES FOR ORGANIZING MENTAL HEALTH ETHICS ROUNDS

NOW THAT THE READER is familiar with the historical and theoretical aspects of ethics in mental health practice, a more practical issue must be addressed: How does one teach mental health ethics? To answer that question, this chapter examines the possible goals of instruction in this area, the variety of approaches taken to the teaching of mental health ethics, and the use of case-oriented material, which the authors have found to be especially useful in the clinical mental health setting. Given the sparseness of the literature on teaching mental health ethics and the commonalities with pedagogic efforts in biomedical ethics as a whole, the works in these areas are cited interchangeably. The subsequent section of the book provides sample case materials that can be employed for case-oriented learning and teaching.

GOALS OF TEACHING MENTAL HEALTH ETHICS

There is widespread agreement among those who teach professional ethics that one goal must serve as the predicate to all others in this discipline. That goal is to heighten the sensitivity of trainees and clinicians to the ethical dilemmas they are likely to confront in routine clinical practice (1–7). In the words of Clouser, "One of the most surprising phenomena about students and professionals is their inability to recognize moral problems as such" (8). Yet, unless the participants in an ethics program begin by acknowledging the relevance of the material to be discussed to their own professional lives, motivation and interest will evaporate, and any more elaborate objectives will remain unfulfilled. Although this objective is usually called "heightening sensitivity", or "consciousness-raising" these terms are deceptive because they suggest that what is involved is merely an alteration of the threshold at which ethical problems are perceived. A more fundamental transformation is often at stake. Participants must learn to reconceptualize the nature of clinical conundra, transforming what were previously defined as technical issues to be resolved by close applications of scientific knowledge and clinical theory into ethical issues that must be addressed in very different ways. Reformulating the initial goal of an ethics program in this way – emphasizing the need to provide new paradigms of thought – better conveys the obstacles that must be overcome in the teaching situation.

The second widely agreed-upon goal of professional ethics programs is to provide participants with a framework for making decisions when ethical issues arise. Numerous aspects of such a framework have been suggested, but the three most essential elements appear to be making professionals aware of ethical theory relevant to the issues they must face, helping to clarify professionals' own values in regard to these issues, and providing an actual model for the resolution of competing values (1–11).

The first component of a framework for decision making – familiarity with relevant ethical theory – may meet with the most resistance from trainees and clinicians. Having worked hard over many years to acquire a clinically oriented approach to the problems they confront (or being in the process of doing so), clinicians will be understandably reluctant to abandon the comfort of their own theories, whose nuances they have explored, for the unknown benefits and possible risks of an entirely different view of the world. There is, in addition, a perception, not wholly unwarranted, that much ethical theory is dry, difficult to understand, and, worst of all, muscle-bound when the clinician is confronted with the need for action. Why compel the clinician to face, even in part to master, this foreign world?

The answer is that, like the novice driver who must learn the meaning of road signs before he or she is competent to navigate the highways, the novitiate in clinical ethics must learn the markers of the terrain. One can, of course, piece the issues together for oneself, labeling the more significant elements idiosyncratically. Such an approach, however, makes it difficult to communicate with others who face similar problems. "Lacking moral distinctions and terminology, (clinicians) are understandably reluctant to take up moral topics with colleagues or patients" (10). Further, the effort that goes into reflecting about the basic aspects of a problem, which may have already been well worked out by others, could be more profitably redirected into a consideration of the fine points of the case at hand. An elementary excursion into ethical theory rewards the clinician many times over by simplifying the task of dealing with ethical issues.

The importance of the second component of the framework – helping clinicians to clarify their own values – should be evident, above all, to mental health professionals. The psychoanalysts have taught us that unacknowledged impulses do not lie dormant in the unconscious, but work their way to the surface in often surprising forms, distorting our behavior and impairing our exercise of conscious control. Thus, the clarification of one's own values can be seen as an important prerequisite to any meaningful change in decision-making patterns. This approach has additional benefits. Many mental health clinicians act, as do all people, on the basis of values they believe to be deeply held, but whose roots they have never explored and whose primacy they have never challenged. The result may be an unwarranted arrogance about the superiority of their own approaches to moral issues (10). When forced to defend their values,

> [s]tudents discover there is seldom one clear and distinct moral answer. They learn more carefully to distinguish among shades of grey.... They see that opposite lines of action are equally moral; but, in understanding the conceptual structures of this opposition, they are more apt to resolve such an instance intelligently and compassionately.... Dogmatism tends to break down, and the complexity of the issues are fully appreciated. These all are part of moral maturity. (9)

The third essential aspect of a framework for decision making is by far the most difficult to convey: a model for the resolution of the competing values that the sensitive clinician is bound to recognize in every complex ethical problem. In fact, the very statement of this goal is misleading because it implies that a single, teachable approach exists to this difficult task. Perhaps it would be more accurate to talk of multiple models for resolving competing values and to recognize the three components that all models must share: (1) a belief that it is possible to decide on action in the clinical setting despite the presence of competing interests (which takes us out of the realm of armchair philosophizing); (2) an ordering of moral values such that some can be considered more important than others; and (3) an insistence that some moral values (e.g., the wrongfulness of wantonly taking a human life) must be above the process of compromise, so that when present they must always take precedence.

Nor can these models be taught in any traditional sense. The process of grappling with ethical conflicts must be demonstrated, and then experienced by the student before he or she can master or even feel comfortable with its use (12). This implies an iterative process, over a period of time, in which the participant is able to experiment with a variety of approaches to resolving competing issues.

Goals in addition to those just discussed have been suggested for teaching programs in ethics, but they are of less universal applicability. Some programs, especially those designed for trainees, have developed multiple objectives that relate to the metaprinciples of ethical theory, such as, "students should understand historical patterns in psychiatric care ... which may have contributed in various ways to current ethical standards and/or particular moral dilemmas ... students should understand the basic principles involved in the psychology of valuing and in moral development" (7). Although this type of approach may be valuable in developing a heightened appreciation of the evolution of ethical standards, many programs might choose to focus more on the practical aspects of applying ethics to the clinical situation.

Other ethics teaching groups are more concerned about the impact of the training they offer on participants' behavior, suggesting, for example, that participants should not only recognize their own values, but "be prepared to take responsibility for shaping some part of the health care system in accord with these values" (11). This goal, of course, is itself the expression of a moral position: that one should feel obliged to alter perceived injustice. Again, not every clinician or program will embrace such an ideal; a justifiable alternative may be to see the obligations of professionals extending only to those with whom they are in immediate contact, their own patients or clients, rather than asking them to promote systemic changes.

The goal of teaching mental health ethics need not be to breed a generation of reformers.

On the other hand, programs that focus solely on providing knowledge, as opposed to stimulating action, are probably more appropriate for the undergraduate classroom than the mental health facility. Ruddick proposes that the goal of training in ethics should be to produce "discursive moral competence," by which he means the "ability to discuss in appropriate moral terminology a variety of routine and rare cases" (10). Fluency in moral terminology may be a desirable side effect of teaching programs in ethics, but it seems unduly pedantic to propose discursive competence as a major goal of such training.

Finally, there is the problematic issue of whether teachers of professional ethics should aim at producing "better" – that is, more moral – clinicians. Goldman and Arbuthnot, working with the model of moral development proposed by Kohlberg, designed their medical ethics program to help participants move to a higher level of moral reasoning than they now occupy (13). As one might expect, this approach has engendered controversy (14). Many ethicists shy away from the implication that their efforts should be directed toward perfecting the moral functioning of their students. They fear, probably correctly, that human motivation and behavior are sufficiently complex that a course in professional ethics is unlikely to lead to dramatic changes in either. What is even more fundamental, they are uncomfortable, in an age of moral relativism, about identifying morally preferable outcomes. Much of the literature on teaching professional ethics contains disclaimers stating that "there is no reason to think that studying ethics will motivate moral behavior any more than studying aeronautics would inspire one to become a pilot" (9). Indeed, unless our society develops a better consensus on moral issues, it seems preferable to eschew normative outcome goals and focus instead on improving the quality of the decision-making process.

APPROACHES TO TEACHING MENTAL HEALTH ETHICS: AN OVERVIEW

Given the diversity of the possible goals of professional ethics programs and the settings in which they have been conducted, it should not be surprising that various approaches have been taken to teaching this material. Three categories of approaches can be outlined: lectures and seminars, case-oriented sessions, and a mixture of the two. Some teaching programs have emphasized traditional lecture and seminar presentations (7, 14–16). In general, efforts of this sort have been directed at students in professional schools who are still involved in regular classroom instruction and therefore are more likely to attend formal sessions. Those programs that stress the communication of specific information related to ethics – such as metaethical theories and the history of professional ethics – tend to employ the lecture and seminar format.

Even within this format, a variety of techniques has been used. One brief ethics course for medical students during a psychiatric clerkship offered sessions on definitions of morality, moral development, paternalism, and the doctor–patient relationship (7). Other courses have addressed similar issues by utilizing excerpts from great works of literature as starting points for discussion (14). Rather than address a large number of ethical issues, some programs have chosen to focus on a single concern – for example, dealing with dying patients – in great depth and with a consideration of related subjects (16). A particularly interesting approach, used for allied health students, has been to introduce decision exercises, which force students to stretch the boundaries of their ethical reasoning, as they must do, for example, in conducting a cost–benefit analysis of possible options in a given situation (15).

The advantages of formal lecture and seminar courses in mental health ethics are obvious. They allow intructors to present ethical theory and other important background material in a structured sequence, so that participants can gain a comprehensive overview of the topic. At the same time, this method gives rise to substantial problems. Many professionals who have completed their classroom training, including advanced professional students, residents, and those who have been in practice for some time, are reluctant to sit through a series of lectures, particularly if the material being presented does not seem to have direct bearing on their practices. In the absence of the compulsion that can be exercised over students, trainees and professionals tend to avoid formal sessions on ethics.

Recognition of this problem has led to a general acceptance of case-oriented teaching for mental health and biomedical ethics courses, especially in clinical settings (1, 3–5, 17–23). With this model, cases drawn from the current caseload, past experience, or published sources provide the basis for an introduction to a particular ethical issue (or set of issues) and the jumping off point for a consideration of alternative approaches. Programs valuing skill in manipulating ethical concepts and the application of principles to clinical practice often utilize a case-oriented format.

As will be discussed in greater detail below, case-oriented ethics presentations can vary widely in their particulars. Some facilities hold "ethics rounds" – formal conferences in which cases are presented and then discussed by participants. These rounds can be open to the general institutional staff or even the public, or restricted to members of a particular clinical unit (20, 21). Alternatively, a classroom setting may be used in which cases are supplemented by additional readings and other instructional techniques are used to encourage participants to consider a number of potential options (17–19). Some programs shun the formality of a conference, preferring to set aside some daily patient rounds – during which the management of newly admitted cases is discussed – specifically to address ethical issues (23).

The popularity of case-oriented approaches testifies to their success in overcoming the barriers created by formal didactic sessions. By presenting ethical conflicts as they are most often encountered by clinicians – that is, in association with particular patients, idiosyncratic contingencies, and a demand for immediate action – cases capture the cognitive and emotional attention of trainees and professionals alike. As important as this is, there is no doubt that case-oriented sessions tend to give less attention to the more formal aspects of ethical theory. They depend heavily on the sophistication and imagination of the group to ensure that all possible options are considered, but even then participants may have difficulty transcending the facts of an immediate case to grasp the larger issues and to draw analogies with comparable situations.

It should be obvious from this discussion that, far from competing with each other, formal lectures and seminars and case-oriented discussions each meet needs that may be neglected by the other approach. Several programs have recognized the complementarity of these models and have offered integrated units on ethics that use both approaches (11, 24–26). As Singer notes in explaining the rationale for this combined model, "The case study approach needs to be supplemented by a more systematic discussion of the nature of ethics and the various ethical theories, like utilitarianism and theories based on rights or justice, from which ethical judgments in particular cases can be derived" (24). Integrated approaches are most easily developed in professional school settings: One model was the medical ethics program at Columbia, which combined lecture series, dinner discussions, day-long seminars, case conferences, and full-time internships in medical ethics (26).

THE CASE-ORIENTED APPROACH

As already noted, the case study method has become a cornerstone of professional ethics courses. This section addresses the practical aspects of a case-oriented mental health ethics program.

Organizational aspects. One of the first steps in organizing a case-oriented ethics program is to specify the background needed by the leaders of the sessions and to select the candidates. The literature is replete with papers suggesting that only professional ethicists are qualified to conduct ethics programs; these papers, of course, tend to be written by ethicists. Even among this group, there is a lively debate as to whether ethicists trained in theological schools are more or less qualified for this purpose than ethicists with degrees from university departments of philosophy. Conversely, many clinicians will avow that only someone with the firsthand experience of dealing with patients or clients can understand the complexity of the issues involved in the most problematic cases.

In some ways, both camps are correct: Each brings to the ethics teaching session a background and perspective that the other lacks. Few clinicians are well enough versed in ethical theory to do justice to the finer distinctions that need to be made in case discussions. Similarly, even ethicists who have become familiar with clinical settings lack the feel for clinical issues and the imperatives clinicians experience that a mental health professional is likely to display. The ideal solution, then, is to combine both sets of talents by having an ethicist and a clinician – each as familiar as possible with the other's area of expertise – serve as co-leaders of the sessions.

Effective collaborations of this sort probably depend greatly on the smooth melding of the personalities involved, but certain ground rules can ease that process. Clinicians should not be limited to commenting solely on the technical aspects of the case; ethicists should feel free to move from theory to clinical questions. In an atmosphere of mutual exploration, disciplinary distinctions become less important. But each co-leader – ethicist and clinician – can be relied upon to keep the discussion intellectually honest when his or her field of expertise is involved.

Practically speaking, the initiative for an ethics program in a mental health training program or facility will usually come from trainees or staff, who are generally people with a particular interest in and perhaps some knowledge of ethical issues. It is important at this point to reach outside the facility, if necessary, to recruit an ethicist who can serve as co-leader. Many local colleges and universities have professors in departments of philosophy or theology who have an interest in biomedical or mental health ethical issues. Local clergymen or hospital chaplains with formal training in ethics are additional resources. Summer seminars on ethics and fellowship programs in clinical ethics have provided a pool of persons from which interested facilities can draw.

When leadership arrangements have been completed, attention will turn to the location and target audience for the sessions. Continuing education programs in most facilities offer logical starting points for many ethics programs. Grand rounds or periodic staff conferences can be reserved for the consideration of ethical issues on a regular basis. The advantages of incorporating ethics teaching into a preexisting program include the use of a time slot in which conflicts are minimized and initial access to an audience that can be counted on to attend regularly. Specially scheduled sessions for discussions of ethics can be problematic because of clinical commitments and because of the unfortunate skepticism that still often attends ethics teaching programs. Many clinicians view ethics as irrelevant to their clinical functioning or treat discussions of ethical issues as nothing more than "bull sessions." Yet, these are precisely the people who most need to be exposed to the consciousness raising aspects of ethics programs. In sum, the use of preexisting conference time is highly desirable.

The target audience for the case study sessions will differ from facility to facility, depending in part on the institution's size. Small organizations will hold ethics rounds or discussions to which the entire clinical staff is invited. Although some larger facilities may also follow this model, which is analogous to clinical grand rounds, there are some advantages to using smaller, unit-oriented conferences for the purpose. In large sessions, presentations tend to be more formal, active discussion is difficult, cases may have to be disguised to protect identities, and participants may be more reluctant to confess their uncertainties about the way they handled or would have handled the case. In smaller groups, in contrast, participants are more relaxed, attendance is often maximized, many participants may already be familiar with cases drawn from actual experience, and interchange among all attendees is facilitated. Ethics programs geared to individual units of a mental health organization can rotate on a weekly or monthly basis, returning periodically to each setting.

The cases that will serve as the basis for discussion can be selected in one of two ways: from the caseload of the participants, or from a compendium of cases, such as the ones provided in this book. Each approach has its strong points, although in many programs it may be desirable to combine these options. Cases drawn from the practices of the participants have the advantage of immediacy and relevance. It is difficult to deny that problems with double-agency, for example, can occur when the illustrative case was seen in one's clinic the previous month. Many staff members will be familiar with these cases and eager to explore the issues with which they themselves have had to struggle.

At the same time, a review of recently seen cases, particularly if it focuses on ethical issues, may leave the clinicians involved feeling defensive, as if their behavior is being questioned. Thus they may be reluctant to present all the data or to explore alternative actions to those pursued. Personality clashes among participants may polarize the discussion and turn the session into a battlefield. Of course, skillful leadership often can defuse these tensions, but cases should be screened for the likelihood of such occurrences before they are selected.

The alternative to using cases from the participants' case loads is to draw cases from a book such as this. This approach provides relatively clear-cut factual situations that can be selected to emphasize particular ethical issues. The overall effect, of course, can be somewhat artificial, since "live" cases invariably have related difficulties that complicate the basic issue, but such simplification may be beneficial when ethical, not clinical, questions are the primary focus. The loss of immediacy is balanced by the fact that paradigmatic questions rarely seen in a facility can also be addressed. Finally, in programs with rotating audiences, there may be some benefit in being able to use the same case repeatedly over time. Law school professors, who rely on the case study method for the bulk of their teaching, are able to explore infinite nuances by dint of their familiarity with cases they have taught for many years. Leaders of ethics rounds may derive similar benefits from practice.

Whatever method is used to select the case, it is advisable for the leaders of the session to confer with unit supervisors or appropriate participants at least one week before the date of the session in order to identify the issue to be addressed and the case to be used. This will give the leaders time to prepare a written summary of the case; and to distribute the summary to participants so that they will be able to follow the presentation and their thoughts will be stimulated in the succeeding discussion. (Written summaries of cases from the facility should be collected after the session to prevent needless lapses of confidentiality.) Presenters should be instructed to limit descriptions of clinical facts to the barest elements necessary to convey the important aspects of the case. Presentations should rarely exceed 10 minutes. Advance selection of the case and topic also allows the leaders, if they choose, to make available a case summary and selected readings in a place convenient to participants before the session occurs.

The final organizational issue to be considered is evaluation. Efforts to assess the effectiveness of ethics teaching programs are desirable for several reasons. First, as with all pedagogy, feedback from the target audience can help the leaders modify the sessions to better meet the needs and interests of participants. Second, if many mental health professionals are still skeptical of the value of teaching ethics, evidence that the sessions are useful and appreciated may help to sustain the program. A review of evaluative techniques is beyond the scope of this chapter, but it can be noted that the focus of evaluation should relate closely to the originally conceptualized goals of the program.

Conducting the sessions. Case-oriented ethics teaching sessions ordinarily begin with a presentation of the essential aspects of the case. When a clinician who was involved in the case is present, it is preferable to have that person outline the major clinical issues, concluding with an indication of the ethical problems that were perceived by the treatment team or the clinician at the time or, for that matter, perceived in retrospect. Others who had contact with the case can be asked to contribute additional material, but the entire presentation should be brief; too extended a focus on the clinical details, though familiar and therefore often comforting to participants, often diverts attention from the ethical issues at hand. Even when the case to be discussed is drawn from another source and written summaries are available, someone should be selected to present the case. Oral presentation focuses attention on the salient issues and in its similarity to the usual clinical conference format provides a link for attendees to potentially unfamiliar territory.

Discussion of the case, stimulated by the co-leaders, will usually evolve in a predictable pattern. To begin the discussion, participants can be asked to identify ethical issues they can see in the case. This is a time of discovery for many in the audience, as issues that had not previously seemed problematic to them are seen in a different light. There may be vigorous debate as to whether a particular issue should be considered ethically problematic or something to be dealt with on a clinical basis. As noted previously, the heightened awareness of ethical problems attained through this process is one of the most important goals of ethics training.

The identification of ethical issues will usually be intermingled with participants' exploration of their own beliefs about the issues under discussion. At this point the co-leaders may become more active, challenging the attendees to justify their positions and leading them backward down the chain of justification to the general principles on which their opinions rest. This process should quickly clarify for the group that differences over the immediate issue reflect less overtly held values about the nature of ethically desirable outcomes. For example, a discussion of the right of the mentally ill to refuse involuntary treatment will usually lead to a consideration of the relative value of autonomy versus paternalistic beneficence.

Here the presence of a co-leader with formal training in ethics becomes especially valuable. When core principles underlying participants' beliefs are identified, it is very useful to take some time to sketch out the theoretical background. In the case of treatment refusal, this may mean a brief elaboration of the value of autonomy in Western thought, philosophical attempts to define the justifiable limits of paternalism, and a sense of how these factors have been integrated historically. There is a delicate balance here between providing sufficient information to ensure that the discussion will proceed usefully and converting the session into an academic discourse on philosophical theories. Leaders will need to experiment with the amount of formal presentation that can be accommodated in the case-study format. Of course, this can be supplemented with readings assigned before the session, with references for participants who are interested in following up on their own, or with a special session to be held subsequently in which a formal introduction to the relevant ethical principles is provided. Problems in attracting clinicians to formal didactic sessions are greatly reduced when interest in them is generated by the group itself, as members come to perceive the need for additional information to help resolve the issues at hand.

The next step, as the session nears its conclusion, is to attempt to achieve some resolution of the issue. Given the view of many people that ethics is of no practical use because all positions are equally correct, it is important to demonstrate to the participants the progress they have made. Leaders should be able to point out that some positions have been rejected by the group and that a limited number of options remain. During some sessions, groups will reach a rough consensus on the issue; that should be noted, although the leaders will always want to challenge a consensus that has been achieved at the cost of ignoring important countervailing values.

When the participants themselves are having trouble attaining closure on the issue, the co-leaders may want to model possible solutions. Particularly in the early sessions in a facility, clinicians may need to see that competing interests must be balanced, but this does not imply that no action is possible. Of course, there will often be cases in which the best resolution is a recognition that none of the current options are desirable. This may suggest the need to alter the existing system or to add to available resources. Participants should come to recognize the interplay between ethical quandaries and reality-based limitations: Ethical issues per se (e.g., the need to triage cases when insufficient resources exist to treat all in need) may disappear when resources are increased. However, to the extent that an increase in resources in one area may adversely affect another area – a frequent occurrence as limited mental health dollars are shifted among competing groups – that solution in itself may bring to light another set of ethical concerns.

A word should be said about special techniques that may promote discussion. Initial presentations may be supplemented by live or videotaped interviews (with permission, of course) of the patient, or of those who may be affected by the decision. The feelings of family members who have been caring for a mentally ill relative, only to see him deteriorate when he is permitted to refuse medication, may serve as a vivid counterpoint to arguments about patients' rights to autonomy. Optimally, videotape or film presentations should be sufficiently balanced so as not to bias the discussants to the extent that opposing points of view cannot be considered.

Special decision-making exercises might also be included, such as those described by Francoeur (15). These can range from techniques in which participants are asked to make sequential decisions based on cumulative disclosures of information, which may highlight the data on which decisions turn, to written exercises in which all possible options are listed and perhaps ranked. Role playing may also be employed to help participants model actions and subsequently discuss their reactions to their behavior.

Pitfalls to be avoided. The first pitfall that the novice organizer of a case-oriented ethics program should beware of is the tendency to view the preceding description of the unfolding of a session as a blueprint to be followed without deviation. Experience with a variety of groups suggests that, depending on background, composition, and setting, the dynamic aspects of group functioning at ethics rounds will differ substantially. Some groups will prefer a more

organized, intellectual approach, with a great deal of formal presentation; others will value free-flowing discussion and will resist efforts
by the co-leaders to impose structure. Some cases will generate intense emotion and involvement; others will require strenuous efforts
to engage the group. Groups may break up into factions insisting
on diverse and contradictory approaches to the ethical issues. Or
they may unite in a common position, resisting the leaders' attempts
to have them consider alternative positions.

Flexibility of approach is a key to effective group ethics discussions. Although the co-leaders will ordinarily meet in advance of a
session to map out the likely flow of the session and the points that
should be addressed, rigid adherence to a preformed plan will defeat
the purpose of the program. If participants are to be encouraged to
reflect on their own values and to experiment with new ways of
conceptualizing and resolving issues, leaders must be prepared to
move with the ebb and flow of the session, digressing to consider
related issues, for example, or focusing an entire session on the one
topic in a case that has captured the group's interest. Leaders with
formal group experience may also find it useful to comment on the
dynamics of the discussion, thereby shedding new light on how
ethical decisions are made. A group's angry denial of the relevance
of a particular factor to the ethical analysis may suggest that the
factor stirs up strong emotions that covertly influence judgments about
the issue. Mental health professionals should be comfortable with,
and capable of making use of, comments of this sort to enhance their
understanding of the origins of their own values.

Group therapists, and experienced teachers, will already be aware
of other pitfalls that may arise. Some participants may attempt to
dominate sessions, especially when they have strong feelings about
the issue under discussion, and may deny the possibility of other
approaches. Participants who maintain, in a show of righteous rage,
that further discussion is useless need to be asked firmly to listen
respectfully to the opinions of others and then perhaps to reconsider
the certainty with which they hold their positions. On occasion the
group as a whole may unite to affirm that only a single position is
worth consideration, and therefore further discussion is moot. This
premature resolution should be challenged by the leaders in an ami-
able spirit that concedes the group may be right, but asks it, as long

as the time has already been set aside for the session, to consider what others might have to say about the issue. In time, such a group may come to understand the fear of moral ambiguity that leads it to embrace an absolutist position.

Countertransference problems can also arise in the conduct of a discussion of ethics. Leaders may positively reinforce comments that echo their beliefs about a subject, as opposing positions are undercut. Their biases may also be reflected in whom they choose to call on during the discussion. Needless to say, indications of favoritism will be rapidly perceived by the group, poisoning the atmosphere of free interchange. People are, of course, pleased to see others adopt their views, so that this process, in its more subtle forms, is difficult to prevent. One useful technique is for the co-leaders to discuss with each other in advance of the session their positions on the issues in order to identify biases that exist. Co-leaders then can be alert to evidence that their colleague's biases are influencing the discussion and can intervene accordingly. When leaders have staked out strongly held positions and doubt their ability to be objective, they may want to inform the group of their stance at the beginning of the discussion. By the same token, if a co-leader chooses, as is often appropriate early in a session, to avoid giving his or her position on the issue in favor of promoting discussion from the audience, that should be explained later to the group as a deliberate choice made for pedagogic purposes. If such an explanation is not offered, there is a risk the group might perceive the leader as "above" worrying about the value conflicts he or she is encouraging the group to consider.

Another form of favoritism that can arise is unique to the mental health setting, in which participants from several disciplines are likely to be present. Some disciplines may be seen, by leaders or participants, as having a superior position in the facility's hierarchy (e.g., psychiatrists or doctoral-level psychologists). This may make the leaders or other members of the group reluctant to challenge these participants' opinions. Since disciplinary biases often color ethical judgments in mental health, this deference may preclude full consideration of the issue. Leaders should beware of such tendencies, being willing themselves, if necessary, to suggest views that counter those of the group's higher-status members.

The leader of a case-study session should also try to prevent ethics rounds from becoming "legal rounds." Given the strong and understandable desire for some guidepost when considering difficult ethical conflicts, participants often inquire about legal requirements that may mandate a particular outcome of an issue. Instead of trying to resolve the tension between confidentiality and the desire to protect others from harm, for example (which is present when a patient threatens to harm a third party), the group may ask the leaders insistently to tell them what the law is on the subject. Once legal rulings are introduced, participants may see the issue as closed and their behavior predetermined.

To avoid this outcome, it is often desirable to note at the beginning of a session that the case under discussion may raise legal issues, but that these will not be addressed this day. (Alternatively, if one of the leaders is aware of the law on the subject, he or she may offer to share that knowledge with the participants at the end of the session.) The leaders should point out that the law is a dynamic construction, often reflecting an evolving moral consensus. Thus, discussions such as those that take place in an ethics session may ultimately come to determine the shape of the law. These cautions may need to be repeated in the course of a session when the temptation to avoid difficult ethical issues by turning to the law arises again.

A final pitfall to be aware of is that ethical issues may be used to screen clinical countertransference issues or to obscure social or political questions. Just as these may become the focus of discourse in an effort to avoid confronting underlying value conflicts, so a premature insistence on reducing a clinical dilemma to a "question of ethics" must be guarded against.

CONCLUSION

This chapter has offered a practical guide to the organization and conduct of ethics rounds and has reviewed the goals of teaching mental health ethics. The next section of this book offers extensive case descriptions, with discussion questions and references, that can be used as the basis of an ethics teaching program.

References

1. Abrams, N. (1979). Teaching medical ethics. *Teaching Philosophy,* 2:309–318.
2. Editorial. (1981). Medical ethics and medical education. *Journal of Medical Ethics,* 7:171–172.

3. Fleischman, A. R. (1981). Teaching medical ethics in a pediatric training pro-
    gram. *Pediatric Annals, 10*:411–413.
4. Bloch, S. (1980). Teaching of psychiatric ethics. *British Journal of Psychiatry,
    136*:300–301.
5. Thompson, I. E. (1981). Teaching of psychiatric ethics (letter). *British Journal
    of Psychiatry, 137*:302.
6. Thung, P. J. (1981). Introducing medical students to ethical issues. *Medical
    Education, 15*:79–84.
7. Salladay, S. A. (1981). Teaching ethics in the psychiatry clerkship. *Journal of
    Medical Education, 56*:204–206.
8. Clouser, K. D. (1980). *Teaching bioethics: Strategies, problems, and resources.* Has-
    tings-on-Hudson, N.Y.: The Hastings Center.
9. Clouser, K. D. (1973). Medical ethics courses: some realistic expectations. *Jour-
    nal of Medical Education, 48*:373–374.
10. Ruddick, W. (1983). What should we teach and test? *Hastings Center Report
    13*(3):20–22.
11. Keller, A. H. (1977). Ethics/human values education in the family practice
    residency. *Journal of Medical Education, 52*:107–116.
12. Michels, R. (1981). Training in psychiatric ethics. In S. Bloch & P. Chodoff
    (Eds.), *Psychiatric ethics.* Oxford: Oxford University Press.
13. Goldman, S. A. & Arbuthnot, J. (1979). Teaching medical ethics: The cognitive-
    developmental approach. *Journal of Medical Ethics, 5*:170–181.
14. Moore, A. R. (1977). Medical humanities: An aid to ethical discussions. *Journal
    of Medical Ethics, 3*:26–32.
15. Francoeur, R. T. (1983). Teaching decision-making skills in biomedical ethics
    for the allied health student. *Journal of Allied Health, 12*:202–209.
16. Thompson, I. E. (1981). Learning about death: A project report from the Edin-
    burgh University Medical School. *Journal of Medical Ethics, 7*:62–66.
17. Abeles, N. (1980). Teaching ethical principles by means of value confrontations.
    Psychotherapy: Theory, Research, and Practice, 17:384–291.
18. Wells, K. B., Hoff, P. A., & Benson, M. C. (1984). A medical ethics tutorial
    program. *Journal of Medical Education, 59*:433–435.
19. Jellinek, M., & Parmelee, D. (1977). Is there a role for medical ethics in post-
    graduate psychiatry courses? *American Journal of Psychiatry, 134*:1438–1439.
20. Levine M. D., Scott, L., & Curran, W. J. (1977). Ethics rounds in a children's
    medical center: Evaluation of a hospital-based program for continuing education
    in medical ethics. *Pediatrics, 60*:202–208.
21. Appelbaum, P. S., & Reiser, S. J. (1981). Ethics rounds: A model for teaching
    ethics in the psychiatric setting. *Hospital and Community Psychiatry, 32*:
    555–560.
22. Self, D. J., & Lyon-Loftus, G. T. (1983). A model for teaching ethics in a family
    practice residency. *Journal of Family Practice, 16*:355–359.
23. Carson, R. A., & Curry, R. W. (1980). Ethics teaching on ward rounds. *Journal
    of Family Practice, 11*:59–63.
24. Singer, P. (1977). Can ethics be taught in a hospital? *Pediatrics, 60*:253–255.

25. Veatch, R. M., & Gaylin, W. (1972). Teaching medical ethics: An experimental program. *Journal of Medical Education, 47*:779–785.
26. Veatch, R. M. (1972). Teaching medical ethics: Helping medical students face ethical issues. *Hastings Center Report, 2*(1):10.

CASES IN
MENTAL HEALTH ETHICS

I

INFORMED CONSENT, COMPETENCY, AND INVOLUNTARY TREATMENT

GIVING IN TO THE PATIENT

When should the patient's views of treatment take precedence over those of staff?

A 52-year old married woman, whose paranoia has been reasonably stable for 18 years, lives with her husband and a niece. Her only psychiatric hospitalization occurred 2 years ago when she was treated with antipsychotic medication. It is not clear what benefit, if any, she obtained from the medication, but she developed a feeling of "heaviness" in her right leg about that time, which she attributed to it. She has since been quite unwilling to take medication.

Two days before the present admission, the patient's home was raided by the police, who were under the mistaken impression that it was a hangout for an escaped drug dealer. The patient was quite shaken by this experience. She became agitated and much more delusional than usual, particularly about her family as well as people in the neighborhood. Although the admission form alleges that she threatened and kicked her husband and niece, it is unclear whether she was ever actually aggressive toward them. They may have fabricated this story to ensure that she would be admitted to the hospital. However, it is clear that she was quite agitated, taking off her clothes repeatedly, and having difficulty getting to sleep. She was evaluated the day following the police raid and was thought not to be committable at that point. But the following day, after a sleepless night, the family obtained an order for commitment.

Since admission, the patient has consistently refused medication. She has not been terribly agitated unless confronted directly with the falsity of her delusions. She has refused any contact with her family. The doctor in charge of her care wants to treat her with medication in the hope of controlling her agitation and diminishing the frequency of her delusions.

Questions

(1) What, in general, are the conditions that would lead psychiatric staff to treat patients despite their wishes?

(2) Does this case fit into that list of conditions?

(3) What are the harms and goods of forcing therapy on this patient?

(4) What are the harms and goods of following the patient's wishes?

(5) What ethical ideals bound the concept of a "right to refuse" therapy?

(6) Are there any significant ethical obligations that the staff should hold toward the family in this case? For example, how strongly should their views of what to do be taken?

(7) Should one consider the additional resources (e.g., prolonged hospitalization) that might be used if the patient's requests were honored? What if the projected period for hospitalization were six weeks without medication and one week with it? What if it were one year without medication and one month with?

(8) How would your answers change if there were empty beds on the unit? If it were filled to capacity?

(9) What if the patient had a sister who, when treated with antipsychotic medication for a similar condition, developed tardive dyskenesia (an involuntary muscle spasm) that did not improve when medication was discontinued?

(10) What if this sister had committed suicide when she was in a similar state, was hospitalized, and refusing medication?

THE RIGHT TO FEEL GOOD

Administering therapies whose "success" is linked to suffering.

The patient was a 29-year-old woman from a prominent local academic family who began experimenting with drugs in her early teens. What followed was an extended period of drug use, prostitution to support it, and a gradual irreversible deterioration of her ability to use cognitive skills, secondary to her massive use of hallucinogens.

For the past 5 years, the patient had been a "street" person, keeping only occasional contact with her estranged family. This hospitalization took place when the patient threatened her father and the police were called.

The patient was placed in a psychiatric hospital, where she was found to have delusions of grandeur and to be in a psychotic but euphoric state. In a structured interview it became clear that the patient's euphoria and psychosis served as a means of avoiding contact with the excruciating but unconscious suffering that she would feel if she allowed herself to become aware of how far short she had actually fallen of her own and her parents' hopes and aspirations. She continued to refuse medications, telling the resident physician, "I'm happy now, I don't want to come down." The resident was faced with this dilemma: To get better, the patient had to pass through a phase of feeling far worse; and even when no longer psychotic she would still face a permanent cognitive loss secondary to her drug use. At the same time, there was no guarantee that her wish, her reality anesthesia, would last long. She was paying a price in terms of being able to function as an autonomous person, and when the reality would finally "hit" her, it might do so in less supportive circumstances – she might "crash," for example, be alone, feel helpless, and attempt suicide.

Questions

(1) Many people in our society consider the pursuit of happiness to be a right. Is happiness itself a right? Is this right in jeopardy in the above situation?

(2) In deciding whether to intervene in the real world, should the clinician weigh equally a patient's conscious and unconscious suffering?

(3) The surgeon operating on an inflamed appendix makes the patient worse for a time (i.e., a hole is made in the abdomen) before making the patient better (removing the appendix and sewing the patient up). Is the issue here comparable? Explain.

(4) Given the medical principles of "first, do no harm," and "try to alleviate suffering," how much suffering may a clinician inflict in the service of doing good? What ethical principles would you use in making this determination?

(5) Given that one "benefit" is the alleviation of *unconscious* suffering, to what degree can a patient who is suffering unconsciously be said to be capable of giving "informed consent"?

(6) How would the risk of an uncontrolled "crash" affect your decision? How immediate would such a risk have to be to justify intervention?

(7) What other data would you wish for to increase the chances that you are making the "right" decision?

DETERMINING COMPETENCY

What factors enter into assessing competency to consent to treatment?

Mrs. B. is an 80-year-old woman with recurrent hospitalizations for alcoholism and depression. She was first admitted shortly after her husband died 12 years ago. Since then each hospitalization has been preceded by a period of withdrawal, isolation, increased drinking, decreased appetite, and sleep disturbance, and the patient has been caring less and less for herself in terms of nutrition and appearance. Her last admission was 3 months ago, at which time she was confused and toxic from hepatic encephalopathy, (a potentially life-threatening impairment of brain function caused by the body's own waste products, which occurs when the liver is so damaged, e.g., by alcohol, that it is unable to metabolize them).

The patient's daughter contacts you stating that her mother once again seems withdrawn and has begun to drink. She wishes her mother would come to live with her but her mother refuses. The patient declines to come for an evaluation.

Questions

(1) Does the threshold for consent for an evaluation differ from consent for treatment? What if the evaluation requires hospitalization? Must the answer be the same for both questions? If the patient's condition worsened markedly – e.g., she stopped eating and became dangerously malnourished – would this change your assessment of the patient's competence? Would it change what you might do? Why?

(2) If on your assessment the patient appears to be nonpsychotic but denies any ill effects of alcohol, in spite of her previous experience, how would this affect your assessment of competency? Are alcoholics competent to decide whether or not to drink? Why or why not?

No - loss control of rational functioning

(3) Compare ethical considerations when assessing the patient's competency to consent to hospitalization, treatment with antidepressants, treatment with electroconvulsive therapy.

(4) What if, at the conclusion of the hospitalization, the patient insisted on returning to live alone and rejected any follow-up care, such as visiting nurse calls? What if the patient's daughter wished to obtain guardianship for the purpose of having her mother live with her? For the purpose of placing her mother in a nursing home?

(5) What if the patient began to speak of it being "God's will" that she die? Would that affect your assessment of competency? What would you do differently?

(6) If the patient had a heart condition, which you believed increased her risk for trycyclic antidepressant medication more than for electroconvulsive therapy, yet she insisted that she be treated by antidepressant medication, would you treat her?

(7) If this patient were forty years younger, would this change any of your previous answers? How?

(8) Discuss the following proposition in relation to this case: "The assessment of competency may be made on clinical grounds alone without reference to an underlying value system."

(9) Discuss the following two views of this case: (a) "The poor woman is just sick and tired of living alone. She has tried her best for 12 years, doesn't feel any better, and so now wants to die. You should have respect for her age and her wishes." (b) "She does not respect her own age, she has been on an extended temper tantrum for the past 12 years; she has not begun to try. She can do better." What are the implicit models of maturity and value inherent in each argument?

SEX AND COMPETENCY

At what point does a therapist's duty to question a patient's competency begin?

Imagine that this case occurs many years before the risks of intrauterine devices (IUD) became known. The patient is a 30-year-old woman outpatient who wants to have an IUD removed. She has a history of bipolar disease (she is manic-depressive with severe mood swings). She is at present a bit "high." She wants to have her IUD taken out because she wants to have "a good time"; she wants to get pregnant this weekend by her boyfriend (who is coming in from out of town) to whom she is not married, and whom she is not telling about the removal of the IUD. She tells you she has decided that if she becomes pregnant, she will keep the baby.

Questions

(1) How would you assess competency to *demand* an IUD removal? Is it a patient's absolute right to have a foreign object removed from her body? Is it ever not so?

(2) How would you respond to the patient's admission that she plans not to inform (or possibly lie to) her boyfriend about the IUD so that he will get her pregnant? Is there a duty for the therapist to warn the boyfriend? What if the law in your jurisdiction would require him to support any child he fathers?

(3) Does the physician have any obligations to the not-yet-conceived fetus?

(4) Assume that the last time the patient had unprotected intercourse she became pregnant, decided to have an abortion, and then asked you not to heed her request for IUD removal in the future, should she become hypomanic. When you tell her of her previous request, she dismisses the reminder. What now?

(5) Would your answers change if the patient was a man telling you that he planned to use a condom with a hole in it in order to impregnate his girlfriend without her consent? What if it were a total stranger? His wife?

Yes – more cause she's deciding to have baby herself

(6) Is there a difference between this patient and a patient who asks you to prescribe some Valium so that he can feel less anxious when making love to his girlfriend? What if he tells you he plans to give her a "mickey" and without her consent impregnate her?

Here he's deciding she'll have a baby.

(7) What would the issues be if one of your patients tells you that he plans to commit adultery unbeknownst to his new spouse? What if the patient is manic? What if the patient is depressed and tells you that he or she feels this will cure the depression as it has in past instances? What if the patient comes from a cultural and religious tradition where multiple wives are accepted?

While both are involved who carries the child matters a big difference

(8) What if the case is taking place in the present when the risks of IUDs are known? Would it make a difference whether or not the patient offered these as reasons for having her IUD removed, but seemingly as an afterthought?

COMMITABILITY AND COMPETENCY

What are the ethical issues in determining the threshold for petitioning for commitment and for questioning a patient's competency to leave the hospital?

The patient is a 28-year-old single female who over the last 9 months has been in a steadily downward spiral. During this period she had three admissions precipitated by depression and suicidality. Not long after one hospitalization she made a *very* serious suicide attempt, overdosing on an antidepressant.

Today, the patient signed a notice requesting discharge within 3 days, stating she planned to leave town – to "start hitchhiking." She had been working up to discharge in any event, with the plan of finding an apartment and continuing in twice-weekly psychotherapy.

There is no evidence of psychosis, and she denies any suicidal intent at the present time. She says the therapist is a very good doctor, feels that he is promising her everything, but that since he is a human being, he is sure to disappoint her at some point. There are thus clear elements of denial and flight present.

Questions

(1) As therapist, you must decide whether to petition for commitment or to discharge the patient against medical advice. What if the patient had a 1 in 1,000 chance of seriously hurting herself, 1 in 100, 1 in 10, 5 out of 10, 9 out of 10? In the next week? In the next month? In the next year? In the next 5 years? How much would the risk without treatment have to increase to justify petitioning? Why? You also feel that, nonetheless, the petition will be denied. What are your obligations to petition in this case? Would your answer change if you felt that the chances of having the petitions granted were less than 1 in 100? 1 in 10? 9 out of 10? Why should or shouldn't that make any difference? Are there any ethical considerations involved in determining your threshold for petitioning?

(2) What if the threat were of the patient hurting her mother instead of herself?

(3) Compare your answers for questions 1 and 2. How could you justify having a different threshold for petitioning if the victim were the patient or her mother? What if the patient had threatened to harm only you – would your threshold be different? Why?

(4) In what sense can this patient be said to be competent to weigh the risks and benefits of discharge?

(5) You feel that your petitioning and the judge's subsequent denial will protect you in case the patient should proceed to harm herself, be- cause you'll be able to feel that you had done the best you could

have. You also feel that this may reduce your risk of liability in case the patient subsequently harms herself. All other things being equal, is it justifiable to act on these feelings? On what basis? How can the act of petitioning be helpful or harmful to the patient herself?

(6) You feel that although the judge may well deny the petition, (i.e., the patient doesn't meet the strict criteria for involuntary commitment) the petition process itself may help to break through the patient's overwhelming denial of her incapacitating anxiety around self-care. Is it ethical to petition (a legal act) for such a therapeutic goal?

(7) Discuss the following proposition: "The assessment of commitability and competency to consent to hospitalization includes the ability to engage in a dialogue resulting in shared decision making." Does this proposition make sense from any of the standpoints of the philosophical positions outlined by our consultants in the case discussed in Chapter 3 on traditions of decision making?

(8) Imagine that a senior clinical consultant and one of our ethical consultants are both available. Whom would you consult first and why? Which questions would you like each to address?

II

CONFIDENTIALITY

KEEPING SECRETS

Are therapists obligated to withhold from patients information they have about their family?

T he patient is a young man in his 20s admitted to the hospital for increasingly disorganized and bizarre behavior. His halfway house is rapidly nearing the limits of its patience with him because of his disruptive lying and stealing; the patient may also be jeopardizing his part-time job by similar antisocial behavior. As the assessment proceeds, the treatment team is struck by the lack of information on this patient, especially concerning his parents and other members of the family. Although the parents live in the same city, they have allegedly cut all ties with the patient and want little to do with him. Similarly, he presents himself as having separated fully from them, and, by inference, the treatment team believes that this again has to do with their reaction to his inappropriate and unmanageable behavior.

After a period of time, a different, deeper perception emerges. It becomes clear that the patient misses his family a great deal, but attempts in a certain sense to "protect" the family from treatment team members by keeping them separated. He almost seems more concerned with their well-being than with himself. It becomes apparent that his recent decompensation is in part caused by the parents' alleged move to a nearby state and his sister's enrollment in a school on the West Coast. The staff soon learn from the parents that they do not wish the patient to know that the move actually took place

Confidentiality

within this very city and that the sister's college is not on the opposite side of the country, but is, in fact, quite nearby. The staff, feeling that the patient should definitely be told such relevant news, communicate this intention to the family. The family reacts with outrage, threatening to drop the patient entirely, to cease all participation in any aspect of his care and placement if the patient is told this information. The staff are torn. They recognize that family involvement is crucial to the patient and to his treatment, but wonder if the patient's long-term improvement, and the ethical standards of his treatment, would be better preserved if he understands the truth.

Questions

(1) What is the basis of, and importance of, trust in the therapeutic relationship?

(2) How important is confidentiality in sustaining such trust and other aspects of the relationship?

(3) How important is "telling the truth" in the therapeutic relationship?

(4) In this case should the therapist have shared knowledge of the family's whereabouts with the patient? Why or why not?

(5) What are the ethical duties of therapists who also work with the patients' families to treat what they hear from the families as confidential data? What allegiance does the therapist have to the family and to the patient? If these allegiances conflict, what principles should guide the therapist?

(6) The family has threatened to leave (which would mean functionally to impair) the treatment if the patient is told about their whereabouts. Suppose the clinic says to the family, "To honor your wish, I won't volunteer information to the patient; but if asked, I won't lie." Defend this approach; attack this approach.

(7) A common ethical dilemma in medicine is whether to tell patients they have cancer. Is the question here of the same order?

(8) Can you think of any situation or circumstance in which *not* giving the patient this information would be useful to the patient?

(9) Suppose the information that the family wants kept secret is that the patient is adopted. Does this change the decisions and the issues? Discuss.

(10) What other information would you wish to know before making your decision? Can you imagine information that you might wish to know but would in some sense be too costly to obtain?

SPILLING SECRETS

The difficulties of balancing confidentiality and harm to others.

The patient is a woman in her 20s on legal probation for assault and battery. She allegedly stabbed someone in the neck. She comes to the hospital voluntarily, with the request, "I need to get myself together."

She says that she feels like two different people, one violent, the other controlled; she is afraid that she will hurt others, especially children; she often hears command hallucinations in the voices of her deceased mother and strangers saying "kill" and "die, die." The patient's relationship to her parents is intensely ambivalent. During the year before her mother died the patient argued with her more than ever. When the mother was ill, the patient refused to help and said once at a family gathering when her mother requested tea, "You make your own," and walked out, slamming the door. The patient's father, who is an alcoholic, remembers only a roughness between them.

Now the patient hears the voice of her dead mother telling her to do things, and she feels compelled to do them, saying, "I never disobey my mother." She also speaks of the entire family joining her *reverting* mother at her own hand – by implication a threat to kill them all. *to child* The memories of her mother, in fact, include moments of closeness *stage before* as well as of abuse and physical beatings. The patient's relationship *problems* with her father is similarly ambivalent. Although quite involved with *started* him emotionally, having spent time following him from bar to bar over long nights to ensure his safety, she expresses both love and disrespect for him and asks staff not to involve him in her case.

The patient's history includes several episodes of violence to herself and others in and out of hospitals; on a number of occasions she has seriously attacked hospital staff. In addition she has made four attempts at suicide and was involved in a single car accident on the day of her mother's death. The patient began drinking at the age of 12 and now considers herself an alcoholic. She feels she cannot control her drinking and claims to have had episodes of loss of control followed by arrests. But the records on these are unclear. She has attended Alcoholics Anonymous, but continues to drink sporadically.

Because of persistent auditory command hallucinations in the form of her dead mother's voice telling her to kill her father, the staff became concerned about a possible duty to warn the potential victim. They drafted a letter informing the father of "a fear she would harm him." When shown the letter, the patient understood the staff's position. She called the father's house and read the letter out loud to her stepmother. The stepmother responded by saying the patient should be locked up and the key thrown away. The patient became convinced that the family would never speak to her again. The staff also insisted on informing the father by telephone, and did so that evening.

Shortly afterward her father called her (having received the letter) and, after a long, intense, highly emotionally charged conversation, her father said "I love you." The patient, much moved, responded with her own declaration of love. Subsequently, although the father was not intensely involved, the patient remained in frequent phone contact with him; the relationship appears to have improved; and the threat of violence is no longer present.

[margin handwriting: Maybe that's all she needed to hear]

Questions

(1) Should the principles of confidentiality and truth-telling be invoked in similar or different ways from the previous case?

(2) How do you weigh the importance of these principles against preventing harm to others? Against preventing harm to the patient?

(3) A recent California court decision (in *Tarasoff* v. *Regents of the University of California*; see Chapter 2) obligates therapists to protect third parties against potential harm from their patients. This puts the therapist in a separate category from most other members of society, who have no such obligation. Is this wise? Why or why not?

(4) In what sense were the decisions taken in this case autonomy-restricting or prompting? In what sense were they paternalistic?

HOW CLOSE IS THERAPEUTIC CLOSENESS?

When personal and professional relationships become blurred.

A 25-year-old woman comes to the ethics committee of the local professional society. She reports that she has been in therapy for depression for 3 years, with a male therapist. She adds that the therapist had given her several gifts, including a book describing women's sexual fantasies. She notes that the therapist encouraged her to use his first name exclusively in her sessions with him. From the beginning, much of the content of the therapy focused on their feelings of mutual attraction, including sexual attraction; in addition, the therapist once used his own extramarital affair as an example to make a point in therapy. She shows the committee letters from the therapist that carry the closing phrases, "Love," "With love," "With deep compassion and loving feelings." Finally she reports that the therapist often patted her shoulder consolingly.

Questions

(1) What would be the "best" and "worst" interpretations or constructions of the therapist's behavior?

(2) Does the patient have a "case"? That is, did the therapist practice unethically – as opposed to practicing unwisely, improperly, ineptly, or failing in some other technical sense? Is this an ethical violation or a demonstration of poor judgment? What guidelines can you construct for distinguishing between the two?

(3) Assume that the patient comes to you for treatment and reports this information to you about her previous therapist. What ethical obligations, if any, do you have? Consider obligations that might impel you both to reveal and to withhold the information you now have. Justify your answer.

(4) In what sense can the patient be said to have had or not to have had a moral responsibility for continuing the relationship if she felt that "it was wrong from the very start"?

(5) Assume the same situation as in question 3 except that the patient reports that this happened to her best friend when being treated by a professional colleague of yours. Again, what obligations, if any, do you have?

(6) Would you modify your answers to questions 3 and 5 if the patient asked you to keep the information confidential?

(7) Would the above answers be modified if the patient was a man and the therapist was a woman? Why?

(8) Imagine that the patient in question reports that the above occurred with her divorce lawyer rather than her therapist. What would you feel obligated to do? She adds that her lawyer told her that dating him would help maintain her morale during divorce proceedings and

that he often recommended sexual relations with him as a "morale booster for trying times." What would your clinical and ethical obligations now be?

(9) Which of the philosophers discussed in Chapter 3 might you consult and for what questions? What additional information might they ask you to obtain? What minimum cost would there be in your obtaining information of this kind from ethics consultants in your hospital? Is the matter of whether to request a consultation an ethical question itself?

THE IMPAIRED PROFESSIONAL

What are the conflicts between respect for a patient's confidentiality and the public good?

A 38-year-old single male is an operating room nurse. He had been hospitalized 3 months ago after lacerating his radial artery with a scalpel. At that time he was diagnosed as having a major depressive disorder and was treated, apparently successfully, with an antidepressant. After discharge, 2 months ago, he was referred for therapy. During the intervening time period he has had mild paranoid ideation, which frequently involved people at work who, he felt, were in some way trying to hurt him. At his regular appointment, it becomes quite clear that he is now actively psychotic. He is having auditory hallucinations of a derogatory nature. He is angry at members of the nursing staff and sometimes has impulses to "lash out" at them, but says that he feels safe around the surgeons, who are "protecting him from the other nurses." He had been taking antidepressant medication every day until about two days ago, when he discontinued it on his own. He accepts a prescription for antipsychotic medication, which he says he might fill. He refuses a suggestion that he be readmitted to the hospital.

Questions

(1) As the treating clinician, what are your ethical obligations? Should the fact that the patient works in a situation where other people's lives are in his hands affect your decision of what to do? Would you feel the same obligations if the patient voluntarily took a leave of absence from work?

(2) Compare this patient with another patient, a commercial pilot with a severe alcohol problem, who is clearly nonpsychotic. Are your duties and options the same?

(3) The patient tells you that his nursing license is up for renewal and he plans to lie in answer to the question asking whether he has been under psychiatric care. What are your ethical obligations? Do they change once the patient is well again?

(4) Imagine that you are intake coordinator for the hospital's Employee Assistance Program and the nurse's operating room supervisor has asked you to see the patient because of some recent absence problems. He has worked at his new job at your hospital for the past month. He did not reveal his past psychiatric history in his job interview. Are you obligated to tell his supervisor what you know? Would your answer change if he accepted your recommendation for hospitalization? What if he accepted your recommendation for hospitalization but only on condition that you kept your interview with him confidential? Does it matter that you are working for the Employee Assistance Program for the purpose of providing "employee assistance and risk management" for the hospital, rather than being paid by the patient or his insurance as his therapist?

WHEN THE VICTIM IS THE SELF

What are the conflicts in respecting the patient's wishes and seeking the patient's good?

The patient is an 18-year-old woman from Italy with no relatives in the United States who has come to study at a nearby university. She has a boyfriend.

This patient recently came to the Student Health Clinic complaining of abdominal pain, at which time she was noted to be extremely thin, weighing 94 pounds. The boyfriend gave the history that the woman was barely eating (only an occasional grapefruit or so) and that she has lost a good deal of weight. The girl did not complain of weight loss at the clinic. In fact, she believed that she was just about the right weight, a common finding in the condition known as anorexia nervosa. The clinic doctor discovers she has an extremely distorted body image.

Questions

(1) Can one ever be said to be competent to starve oneself to death?

(2) Is any intervention by clinic staff called for?

(3) If the patient had family in this country, would this change your sense as to what is the best thing to do?

(4) If you felt that the patient was not committable but in dire need of treatment, would you notify her family in Italy? Would you do so without the patient's permission? Under what circumstances?

(5) Would the patient's medical condition and plans with regard to future weight make a difference in your decision to contact the family? What about other interventions such as involuntary hospitalization or even "forced" feeding? Why? How?

(6) Can you use one of the philosopher's arguments in Chapter 3 to justify the proposition that in the main the questions that need to be addressed are medical? Ethical? Which do you believe? Why?

(7) Compare the ethical issues involved in breaking confidentiality to warn one member of a family that another is contemplating self-harm, as opposed to warning this family member that the other may be dangerous to her. Is the case different if the patient is unpredictably violent and may endanger anyone at any time?

III

TRUTH-TELLING

What to do when suspecting collegial malpractice.

The patient is a 39-year-old male with a diagnosis of chronic schizophrenia. His condition is followed in a Schizophrenia Clinic, where he comes every two weeks for an injection of medication. He has a low IQ, severe character problems, and occasionally develops paranoia, which is well controlled with medication. He sometimes engages in voyeuristic behavior, which diminishes when the dose of medication is increased.

While under this psychiatric treatment, the patient suffered a gall bladder attack and had his gall bladder removed. Two months after the operation, he called on the psychiatrist complaining of increasing pain and difficulties in moving his left hand. He was referred to an internist who found stiffness in his left arm and loss of sensation and muscular atrophy of the fourth and fifth fingers. He was treated with drugs for possible nerve damage for several months, but without improvement.

At this point, the psychiatrist began to question him about when he had first noticed the problem. The patient replied that it had begun about 2 or 3 days after discharge from the hospital. He said that the problem did not interfere with his life, because he was still able to perform basic housekeeping chores and go shopping for his mother, but that he would like to know what is going on. Since the psychiatrist was affiliated with the hospital where the operation took place, a review of the hospital chart by him, including the operative report, was possible without the patient's knowledge. No complications were listed in the report and no note was made of any possibility of injury to the patient's arm. The psychiatrist suspects that injury to the arm occurred during surgery, but fears that sharing this suspicion with the patient may provoke a malpractice suit against the surgeon.

Questions

(1) In general terms, does the psychiatrist have an obligation to ensure that the patient receives the best possible medical care by informing the internist treating the patient of his suspicions concerning the source of injury?

(2) Does the psychiatrist have the further obligation to share his suspicions with the patient? Should he have obtained the patient's permission to review the chart?

(3) Can this patient claim a right to any knowledge that doctors and medical staff may possess concerning his illness?

(4) If the psychiatrist informs the patient's surgeon about his suspicions, what, if any, are the obligations of the latter?

(5) Should there be a hospital policy to deal with such a case? If so, what? What effect should the patient's low IQ have on the actions of the parties in this case?

(6) Should the psychiatrist's actions differ if the patient's paranoia is expressed in a desire "to make someone pay for what has happened to me"? If the patient's history involves numerous lawsuits against authority figures? Threats of violence?

(7) How would the search for the "right" decision be framed by your interpretation of the surgeon's role in "causing" the patient's injury?

(8) Would the fact that the patient was poverty-stricken play a role? Is the last consideration a valid one on clinical grounds? On ethical grounds? What would the philosopher consultants in Chapter 3 have to recommend regarding whether this factor should be considered?

CAN YOU WRITE ME A NOTE?

When is it appropriate for a mental health therapist to enter a controversy involving a patient's social problems?

The patient is a manic-depressive 24-year old dental student who is being treated with lithium. He has had a two-year history of psychiatric disorder, and he has done very poorly in dental school, failing some tests when manic. Most recently he did not pass his examinations in the second year, having repeated the first year previously. He is now suspended from school and being managed on lithium.

It is summer, and the psychiatrist has written a letter to the dental school about the possibility of the patient being readmitted. She has told the patient that perhaps he would do better to wait and begin school in January, even though her letter recommends that he be readmitted in the fall.

After the letter was sent, the patient petitioned the dental school for readmission. The petition was denied, and the patient became deeply troubled. The denial stirred the psychiatrist to try to write the school admissions committee to discuss the matter with them.

Failing to hear from the committee, the psychiatrist went to see the dean. He told her that there had been an error: The school had lost her letter about the patient, and it had never even been considered when his petition was denied.

The dean urged the psychiatrist not to tell the patient what had happened, and suggested that perhaps the matter should be smoothed over in some other way. The patient, meanwhile, was angry and bitter. On the very day of and following the psychiatrist's talk with the dean, the patient told her that he was disgusted with the dental school, and that if he were not readmitted he would sue. The psychiatrist, who had been working with him therapeutically on issues of anger and bitterness, pondered what to do.

Questions

(1) One way to approach this problem is to conceal the facts from the patient to prevent a possible worsening of his psychiatric condition or keep from jeopardizing his prospects for readmission to dental school. Would such a "paternalistic" approach be acceptable?

(2) Another approach would be to give him the facts and help him to cope with them, reasoning that he has the right to know the truth. Would this autonomy-based approach be best?

(3) Should the psychiatrist do nothing, and let the dean and the patient work out the problem?

(4) What other approaches to this problem are possible? What are the ethical issues they raise?

(5) Is this a "medical problem"? How would your answer influence your actions?

(6) Would your answers differ if you were employed as a psychiatrist by the dental school?

(7) The patient tells you he wishes to do "the grown-up thing." Would this influence your decision? How? What sorts of values are implicit in your picture of what it means to be grown up?

HELPING PATIENTS, HURTING OTHERS

Should a therapist help a patient deceive others?

A patient with schizophrenia who is in long-term therapy is able to work at a steady job and considers applying for a promotion. As part of this promotion he would be expected, like any other employee, to take a battery of psychological tests. The patient is fearful about this requirement. He is worried about what would inadvertently surface, especially his long history of emotional disturbances, of which his employers are allegedly ignorant. If the tests might reveal these facts, he would forgo them and not apply for the promotion; if they would not, he would seriously consider the application.

The patient asks if the therapist would be willing to administer a comparable battery of tests to the patient and review the results with him; this would give the patient a basis for making the decision about whether to go through with the application process.

Questions

(1) Given that patients with mental illness find it extraordinarily difficult to get and hold jobs – not the least because of the information they must often reveal about their psychiatric histories – advice and assistance in employment and rehabilitation are commonly given by therapists to patients, including "mock interviews" with simulated employers. Is the case above different? How or how not?

(2) Should concern for the patient's employer enter into the therapist's decision? Even if the patient has no intent to deceive, is his request fair to his employer? In effect, the patient is being pre-tested or "primed" with answers that could conceivably be put to use in deception. Assuming that this was the therapist's actual intent (as did

not seem to be the case here), would that approach find room under the heading of doing everything one can in one's patient's interests? Would knowledge that an employer unreasonably discriminates against handicapped persons affect your answer?

(3) Would your decision be affected by the kind of job to which the patient was being promoted? For example, suppose the job involved some responsibility or risk to a population of people, where the patient's conduct might lead to possible harm?

PAY UP OR CLAM UP

Should failure to pay appropriate medical bills influence an institution's willingness to cooperate in patient care?

The treatment of a child, and secondarily his parents, was terminated at a family guidance center when the family's bill reached $2,000 and the center learned that the family had spent a $400 insurance check that would have covered a part of that expense. The treatment of the child was just about over, and the remaining issues were mostly parental when termination took place. The facility intended to turn over the unpaid debt to a collection agency.

Shortly thereafter, the center's director received a release-of-information form signed by the father for the child's records, in connection with treatment at another facility. The center's director wonders whether, given the family's failure to pay the bill, the institution is obligated to turn the records over to the new treatment facility.

Questions

(1) Does the center have an ethical warrant to refuse to turn over the records to the new facility because of failure to pay the bill, given the fact that the law in this state made the center the owner of the child's records, although the information they contain belongs to the patient?

(2) How much should the welfare of the child count in this case?

(3) Should the institution turn over the records only with an indication of nonpayment included in them?

(4) Are the parents morally entitled to see what is sent? To be told in advance, without asking, that evidence of their failure to pay will be

included? If they object to the nonpayment issue being included and refuse to request the records if it is, should the center's director exclude it?

(5) How much difference would it make if the family were very poor? Very rich? If the center were able to absorb this loss easily?

(6) How should the center respond if the patient's parents return wishing further treatment for the child? For themselves?

(7) Are there clinical circumstances under which telling the child about the parent's failure to pay the bill during the course of therapy could be ethically justified?

EXCISING EVIDENCE

How should a therapist weigh the harms and benefits of deleting material from a psychiatric report?

A therapist who has been working on a fairly regular basis for a public defender was asked to do a "general forensic examination," apparently designed to determine a defendant's competency to stand trial, criminal responsibility, and diminished capacity, and whatever aid for the trial that could be provided. The therapist performed the examination on a man who was facing charges of sexual assault of a child. It turned out, and was included in the therapist's report, that the man had a long history of pedophilia, most of which had never come to the authorities' attention. The therapist saw this information as a legitimate part of the report because he viewed this history as an indication of a significant psychiatric disorder, which might suggest that the court recommend treatment instead of incarceration.

Subsequently, the public defender and the prosecutor agreed to a plea bargain, as a part of which the defense was to turn over all psychiatric and other reports that had been prepared on the case. The public defender contacted the therapist at that point and asked if he would delete from his report the incriminating material that dealt with the defendant's past, undiscovered offenses. The public defender said that the information was no longer relevant to the case. He worried that if the prosecution got hold of that material, it could cause the plea bargain to fall through, since the prosecutor might at that point decide to seek a more severe punishment for the defendant. The therapist asks whether it is legitimate, or as he puts it "ethical," to alter his report in these circumstances.

Questions

(1) In this situation, what are the therapist's ethical obligations to the defendant? What is the nature of the relationship between the therapist and the defendant?

(2) What are the therapist's ethical obligations to the prosecutor, and the state and society he represents?

(3) Is there a general obligation for the therapist to report faithfully in the medical record what is learned of the case, and not to alter it? If so, are there occasions when exceptions should be made to this rule?

(4) What would you do if you were the therapist, and why?

(5) What if the setting were private, the examination performed at the request of the defendant's lawyer, and at the lawyer's expense?

(6) Do any of the philosophical positions discussed in Chapter 3 provide additional views concerning the potential future dangerousness of the defendant? Do any make a difference for you?

(7) What additional information could make a difference? Which values are you subscribing to in saying this? Which philosophers might find these congenial or not?

IV

MANAGING DIFFICULT PATIENTS

HELPING AND HATING

How, ethically, should the intense dislike of a patient by staff be handled?

The patient is a male in his mid-30s whose diagnosis is uncertain. The primary possibilities are chronic manic-depressive illness or schizoaffective disorder. The brilliance of his childhood is reflected in his being able to play the piano at age three. Doted on by his mother, he was the star of his family and was frequently shown off. He had his first psychotic break at the age of 15 while in private school, apparently over the stresses of sexual maturation and various identity issues. He had a number of treatments with electroconvulsive therapy and hospitalizations over a period of several years during which he never achieved independent living.

Ten years prior to the present admission the patient's sister and her husband brought the patient to a different city in an effort to rehabilitate him. He did reasonably well on a new medication and remained out of the hospital until this admission.

The patient's inpatient contact is characterized by numerous medical problems, a profound tendency toward serious regression in the hospital, and a serious inability to use the hospital in any constructive way. He is very demanding, frequently expressing anger toward staff and getting into struggles with the staff over medications, restrictions, and the like.

After 3 months in the hospital, he is discharged at his insistence, but brought back involuntarily only a week later for threatening a fellow resident at the halfway house. During this second admission, the patient is tried on various new medication regimens which, in combination with a strict ward program and intensive occupational therapy, help him to move to more independent living at a halfway house.

But the patient subsequently becomes quite disorganized under the impact of a very serious sequence of stressful events, takes his medications irregularly, is sleeping poorly, threatening people on the street, and visiting the hospital frequently, demanding to be seen and then leaving or yelling so that no conversation could be carried on. The sister calls the hospital numerous times saying she feels that the patient needs hospitalization for stabilization. This is finally arranged. The patient is hospitalized for one day before signing a paper requesting discharge. He is found "not commitable" and is discharged, only to repeat his disorganized behavior. He is placed in a halfway house again (so that at least his medication can be administered regularly) but the behavior persists. He starts fights with people on the street and has to be restricted from the inpatient ward for threatening behavior and inappropriate sexual behavior; he threatens the doctor, the secretaries, and the superintendent. Finally, he is readmitted.

During this time, the patient's sister complains bitterly to social workers, treatment team therapists, and administrators, stating that the hospital is negligent, that the patient is likely to get himself hurt, and that, if anything happened to him, the hospital would be responsible. Although all the people just mentioned are in communication with each other as part of the active treatment program, there is yet a sense of not knowing who is ultimately responsible. The case is reviewed in conference to look at the question of where the ultimate responsibility lay and what could be done with a patient who generates hatred in treatment staff because of his intransigence, resistance, hostility, and, perhaps most fundamentally, his nonresponsiveness to all kinds of modalities of treatment available.

Questions

(1) What are the respective obligations of family and hospital staff to this patient?

(2) What is the relationship between their respective responsibilities?

(3) What circumstances in general might provide ethical justification for

the staff to withdraw from a relationship with this patient and what is the nature of such justification?

(4) What would you do in this case and why (apply the discussion above)?

(5) Can a treatment team help someone whom they hate?

(6) Under what circumstances should a response of hatred be just another clinical problem to be resolved in a way similar to other emotional responses to difficult patients?

(7) Compare this case with the case, "Do Not Resuscitate for the Living" (Chapter VII). Compare the two cases, first in the language of rights and obligations and then in the language of risks and benefits.

(8) Under what circumstances are the staff morally responsible for experiencing hatred toward the patient? Which of the philosophers in Chapter 3 might consider an exploration of the clinical significance of the hatred to be valuable or insignificant from an ethical standpoint? What do *you* think?

WHAT HOME FOR THE VIOLENT?

What level of risk should staff endure in treating dangerous patients?

The patient is a powerfully built woman in her early 30s admitted to a psychiatric hospital on a court order for being uncontrollable at the pre-trial hospital unit at the women's prison. The patient had been hospitalized for assaultive behavior almost continuously since the age of 13, with recurrent admissions to hospitals in three different states. The possibility of temporal lobe epilepsy (a rare cause of violence) was raised as a contributing factor, but treatment with anticonvulsant medications did not diminish her aggression. A number of her symptoms suggested a diagnosis of psychosis, perhaps even childhood schizophrenia, but many different antipsychotic compounds were also found to be ineffective.

During all admissions to various hospitals the patient was a behavioral problem for the staff. At one point she was managed on a locked ward with frequent periods of room confinement and brief periods of seclusion for assaultive behavior. Several serious assaults on staff occurred during one of her hospitalizations when she hit one with a table, struck another, and attempted to stab a third with a knife. One of the hospital staff treating her decided to bring charges against her, and she was arrested and sent to another hospital for an evaluation of her competence to stand trial. The staff at this next hospital were quite exhausted and genuinely frightened of the patient, and some felt that they might prefer to quit or be fired if they were required to treat her.

Negotiations were then started for her transfer to yet another mental hospital. The patient's behavior at that time included banging her head on the seclusion room wall, attempting to grab a court officer's gun so that she could kill herself, numerous incidents of verbal assaults, one incident of her setting her clothing on fire, and other episodes of violence directed not only at the staff but at other patients and courtroom personnel. A wide variety of antipsychotic regimens failed. Psychological testing revealed a low IQ, intense perfectionism, and a life dominated by preoccupations with sadistic impulses, with much fusion of sexual and aggressive imagery. The patient's stories on projective testing indicated that she had probably suffered brutalizing experiences in the past, none of which she was able to communicate, and that she was constantly reliving these, almost as if she had to be wary of their recurrence in the present.

On the current admission, as in the past, the patient proved particularly exhausting, frustrating, and infuriating to the staff. A great deal of this feeling stemmed from the difficulty of distinguishing when or whether the patient was actually in the grip of a psychotic process and when she was really being contentious, provocative, and distressing for her own emotional satisfaction or upon not getting her own way. During the present admission the patient was repeatedly assaultive and threatening and engaged in attempts at self-mutilation (for example, she tried to pierce her eyes on both sides with splinters formed from a tongue depressor). She refused medication as a regular regimen, but received numerous emergency involuntary injections of medication for intermittent assaultiveness. The patient manifested large numbers of primitive behaviors including the smearing and eating of her own feces.

The Department of Corrections made it clear that there was no place for the patient in its system. When the patient ultimately was discharged from the hospital to the court, the judge determined the patient was "not fit to return to the community," and she was returned to the hospital on another court order, a procedure which was believed by legal experts to constitute a possible violation of the patient's civil rights by the court.

Questions

(1) What distinctions can be made between emotionally uncontrollable versus criminal actions? Between the person who will not and cannot control herself?

(2) Given these distinctions, what are the ethical justifications, from a social viewpoint, for confining this patient? For confining her in a mental institution? For confining her in jail?

(3) Compare the ethical justifications the staff might offer in refusing to treat this patient and the ethical justifications for the same decision in the "Helping and Hating" case (Chapter IV).

(4) What ethical justifications might the hospital administration offer for compelling the staff to treat this patient?

(5) What are the obligations of the staff to protect one patient from another? To protect the community at large from a discharged patient? What would you do, and why, when these two obligations conflict, as they do with this patient, who has proven to be violent in *or* out of the hospital?

(6) Is there any other information about the case that you would find valuable in answering the above questions? What values are reflected in your answer? What paradigm of clinical science would you be following?

HIS OWN WORST ENEMY

Short-term perils versus long-term benefits of handling self-destructive behavior.

The patient is a 29-year-old college graduate who was admitted to a psychiatric hospital after a suicide attempt in which he slashed his wrists. In the last year he has had five psychiatric admissions, each precipitated by suicidal ideation and gestures. The central issue in his life has been his separation from and upcoming divorce of his wife of 8 years. The patient's diagnosis is borderline personality; he has a history of many years of multiple drug abuse, including alcohol, hallucinogens and stimulants. In the patient's previous hospitalization, he received therapy for a very brief time and rapidly recompensated, with a marked decrease in suicidal ideation. But the patient's recovery was accompanied by some difficulty in taking his problem seriously and assuming responsibility for his ongoing treatment.

Just prior to this hospitalization, the patient returned to the local area from another part of the country, hoping for a reconciliation with his wife. When it became clear this was impossible, he became despondent, wandered the streets, took impulsive overdoses of antidepressants, and felt he had failed because he had not died. He was then admitted to the hospital, escaped, returned, and was placed on constant observation. While on the ward, he engaged in repeated wrist slashing; despite this, constant observation of him was gradually tapered successfully.

Two months after admission, he began to bang his head violently against the wall of his room, and when he was secluded, against the wall of the seclusion room; he did this, he said, to express self-hatred. This behavior consisted of the patient seating himself with his back to the wall either on the floor or the bed, bending forward at the waist, and slamming his whole upper body backward against the wall, causing a terrific impact from his head against the plaster wall. This intensified over the next 6 months and was occasionally punctuated by additional wrist slashing. The staff working with him had mixed feelings about his management. On the one hand, he was felt to be seriously ill and quite self-destructive both in active terms (such as the wrist slashing and head banging) and in passive terms (such as his refusal to eat at certain times). On the other hand, it seemed that intensive treatment of this patient could demoralize the unit, staff, and patient alike.

The staff struggled with a number of ways of dealing with the patient. They wondered, first, whether engaging the patient in conversation when he became more disturbed would distract him from self-destructive impulses and fill his need for attention. Others argued that the attention was serving as the reward for self-destructive activities and was thus perpetuating this behavior. The struggle over doing something versus doing nothing about the head banging took various forms. Some staff wondered if the patient should be made to take more responsibility by paying for the plaster walls that he was damaging by the violent contacts with his head. Others wondered if he should be provided with football helmets or motorcycle helmets and should be obligated to wear these as protection for his head so that the banging would do less bodily harm. Many staff members believed that responsibility was the crucial variable in a patient like this, and that "curing" him, though representing a reasonable goal, may be less important in the short run than demanding that the patient learn to take responsibility for his actions.

Questions

(1) What degree of self-harm ethically justifies intervention by the clinician? In answering consider compulsive hand washing, failure to use seatbelts, heavy smoking, driving while drunk, head banging, wrist slashing, and suicide. What intervention is ethically justified for each of the above cases and what should be the limits of such intervention?

(2) Is it ethically justifiable to have the patient pay or not pay for the damages mentioned in the case? Would the response to this be any different if the patient were psychotic?

(3) Assume that watching the patient from an arm's length away stops the head banging behavior but ties up one staff member completely, placing other patients on the ward at some increased risk and at some decreased level of care. Ethically justify taking this course, and not taking this course.

(4) The goal that "the patient should be made to take responsibility for his actions" reflects both autonomy and paternalistic value considerations. Discuss. Is there also an implicit model of how "responsibility" cures?

(5) Discuss from the vantage point of each of the four philosopher consultants in Chapter 3 what degree of self-observation would be required for ascription of responsibility? Would you require the same degree of self-observation for ascription of responsibility for praiseworthy acts as for blameworthy ones? Is there any other sense of a responsibility besides praise or blame that is clinically important (e.g., being able to say "this is me")? Is emphasizing this sense truly value-free?

(6) "You are morally responsible for what you *do*; what you *feel* is beyond good and evil." Discuss in reference to this case.

V

PARENTS AND CHILDREN

When is it appropriate for therapists to override parental wishes?

A 9-year-old girl was admitted to the Children's Psychiatric Unit with a history of multiple somatic complaints, refusal to go to school, and in the past year, although not currently, a history of such minor self-abuse as inflicting scratches on herself. The patient evidently had been having trouble for some time, but only recently had the parents agreed to bring her in for psychiatric evaluation. When she does attend school, she does well. She has a 6-year-old sibling who, according to the clinicians in the Children's Unit, has attempted suicide recently, certainly an unusual occurrence in a child that young. In addition, it is reported that prior to admission the patient was sleeping up to 17 hours a day.

Five days after admission the patient's mother called, saying that she intended to take the patient home with her that afternoon. The clinicians at the Children's Unit do not view this family sympathetically. The father was described as withdrawn and anxious, and the mother as anxious with pressured speech. The ostensible reason for their wanting to take the child out of care was that the child's grandmother had just been hospitalized for a bleeding ulcer, and the family wanted to have her back home so that they would not worry about her as well. The clinicians thought that perhaps the real reason they wanted her at home was to care for her younger brother while the mother was off tending to grandmother.

What made this an issue for the unit staff at all was their belief that this child had been subjected to abuse in the past. On her labia and in the perineal area, they found what they considered many signs of old trauma, including something that looked like a scar from a cigarette burn. However, they felt confident that these signs of trauma were at least one year old and maybe older. The child denied any injury or physical abuse, said the scars were always there, and that her mother told her they were present at her birth. The parents had not been confronted about a suspicion of child abuse.

Questions

(1) How should the unit staff act, from the viewpoint of ethics, toward possible evidence of previous child abuse? Assume, as was the case here, that the state's reporting statute is ambiguous about whether suspected previous abuse must be reported.

(2) Should evidence of recent abuse be treated differently from that of past abuse?

(3) How do you weigh the moral warrant of the unit staff in this case, versus that of the parents, to determine what happens to the child?

(4) Is there a role for the state in this case, or should the unit staff and the parents work it out?

(5) Do the staff have any moral obligations to the parents, or solely to the child?

(6) Without the history of a sibling suicide attempt, would your answers be the same?

(7) If the parents themselves admit to having been abused as children, would your level of concern be affected? What if there was a family history of drug and alcohol use?

(8) Review clinical and ethical considerations to understand the conflict the staff is feeling about confronting the parents. In what sense may this be "countertransference" and in what sense may this be "an ethical dilemma?" Can it be both?

DISCOVERING ILLEGAL BEHAVIOR

The dilemmas of a social worker who learns about her patient's violation of the law.

A social worker at a parent-child guidance center had been seeing a woman with two daughters, one 5 years old and one 13 years old.

The 5-year-old is the identified patient. Mother and daughter were referred following Child Welfare's investigations of the mother for child neglect and a judge's order that the 13-year-old be sent to a group home. When the social worker called the patient at home, the 13-year-old daughter, who the social worker knew had recently escaped from the group home, answered the telephone and admitted her identity. At their next session, the mother admitted that she was harboring the daughter, but quickly said that she did not want the social worker to tell anybody about it, particularly Child Welfare. The social worker's agency is encouraging her to tell Child Welfare about the phone call, saying that she has an ethical obligation to report the mother for harboring this runaway child. The worker feels very uncomfortable with this.

Questions

(1) Does the social worker have an ethical obligation to report the mother to Child Welfare?

(2) Would possible evidence that the 13-year-old was being abused by the mother change your view of the social worker's obligation?

(3) Would the possibility of endangering the therapeutic relationship between the social worker and the mother and 5-year-old daughter be a significant enough deterrent to notification of Child Welfare?

(4) Should the social worker have discussed the problem with her colleagues at the guidance center? Does the social worker have obligations to any one else? Why?

(5) Once the authorities at the guidance center have learned of the problem, what are their obligations?

(6) From the viewpoint of ethics, what would you do if you were the social worker?

(7) How would your answer change if you believed that the 13-year-old was at significant risk for drug and alcohol use? What if she previously had been abusing her younger sister repeatedly? What if her mother said to you about the 13-year-old, "I can't live without her"?

(8) As the social worker, what further information would you value in deciding whether the mother was acting responsibly or irresponsibly? How would that help you to act "ethically," "paternalistically," "responsibly," "clinically"? Define these terms. What values and standards are implicit in your definitions?

(9) Is this a situation in which it is either your authority or the patient's mother's? What do you mean by authority?

WHAT DOES IT TAKE TO ACT?

The dilemma of whether responsibility to protect the interests of a child should jeopardize the health of her mother.

The patient, a 12-year-old girl, initially came to a psychiatric out-patient clinic with her mother at the request of the state welfare authorities and because of her teacher's concern over the child's obvious behavioral disturbance.

In the course of the evaluation, it was learned that, although there was no physical abuse and the child was well fed and well clothed, the mother tended to oscillate between being emotionally unavailable to the child during the day and preferring to sleep with the child instead of her husband at night. Psychological testing revealed a severely disturbed child who in all probability was in the midst of a psychotic relationship with her equally severely disturbed mother.

As the evaluation progressed, the mother became frightened that the child would be taken away from her and refused the offer of hospitalization for the child. The staff became divided in this particular case about whether or not to press the issue in court, and initiate action, which, though possibly benefiting the child, might lead to the *mother's* decompensation. What made the decision so difficult was that there was no evidence of overt physical abuse, but rather only subjective clinical and psychological test data of a severely disorganized mother-daughter emotional relationship.

Questions

(1) Since no mother is perfect, after all, what is the ethical justification for pressing in court the issue of hospitalizing this child?
(2) How would your answer change if there was only little risk to the mother's mental health in petitioning the court?
(3) Compare this case to a case of physical child abuse.
(4) Justify leaving the child with the mother in terms of the language of risks and benefits. Justify it in terms of rights.
(5) Would your answer change if the child was much older? Much younger?

(6) How would your answer change if the child showed severe impairment in reading ability on a standardized test? Compare this situation to the child who shows a severe impairment in emotional stability on a standardized test.

(7) Give the ethical justifications for viewing physical, emotional, and cognitive harms as entailing *equivalent* or *differing* thresholds for intervention by clinicians.

(8) On further evaluation the child herself expresses intensely ambivalent wishes. One day she states she wants to stay with the mother, no matter what; another day she says she would rather die than continue to live with her. How would your ethical justifications take these ambivalent wishes into account?

(9) What could an assessment of the child's father contribute to your ethical justification? What values are implicit in your answer? Are the values ethical, social, clinical? How do these differ?

WHEN MOTHER'S RIGHTS AND FETAL INTERESTS COLLIDE

What is the proper role for a psychiatric consultant when a pregnant woman refuses treatment that may be essential to preserve the life of her fetus?

A 21-year-old woman was admitted to an obstetrical service in her 32d week of pregnancy. She was diagnosed as suffering from preeclampsia, a syndrome of unknown cause in pregnancy, marked by elevated blood pressure, kidney malfunction, and the risk of seizures, kidney failure, and stroke in the mother, as well as loss of the fetus. Treatment of a case as advanced as this patient's involves immediate control of her blood pressure with intravenous medications and induction of labor, so that the baby can be delivered before harm occurs. The syndrome resolves with the birth of the fetus.

When this patient was admitted, however, she refused any treatment, including the placement of an intravenous line and even a pelvic examination. Initially she related the reasons for her refusal to her "fear of needles," as both treatment of her hypertension and induction of labor would have required intravenous lines. Later, she was extremely distraught, nearly "hysterical," and offered no reason at all for her refusal. Nonetheless, during her calmer moments, she exhibited a good understanding of the nature of her condition, the possible consequences of refusing treatment, and her physicians' recommendations.

A psychiatric consultant who attempted to determine what lay behind the patient's refusal of treatment discovered that, when she married, the patient had converted to her husband's religion, which required her to stay at home and shun contact with society. They planned ultimately to return to the husband's homeland, when he completed his studies in this country. The psychiatrist's hypothesis that the patient was ambivalent about her marriage and the unborn child that would cement it was contradicted by the husband, who reported that the patient was eager for her baby's birth and had been making extensive preparations for the child's arrival. It was also discovered that the patient and her husband had no hospitalization insurance; thus they would be paying for the care she received out of their own pocket.

All attempts to explore the patient's feelings about her pregnancy and marriage over a 5-day period, or to offer support in resolving the family's impending financial difficulties, were rebuffed. The patient's mother soon appeared on the scene, confirming that the patient had had a life-long fear of hypodermic needles. Efforts to obtain a hypnotist, so that she might accept an IV while in a hypnotic trance, were unsuccessful. The obstetricians, meanwhile, had come to the conclusion that immediate intervention was now crucial to saving the life of the fetus, and perhaps the patient as well.

The patient's obstetricians told the psychiatric consultant that they would be willing, on the advice of the hospital attorney, to proceed with induction of labor over the patient's objections if the consultant would certify the patient as incompetent. The consultant, while recognizing the importance of prompt treatment, felt that this patient, who was able to express her desires and understand the nature of her situation and the likely consequences of different courses of action, would in fact be considered competent by a court. Although the patient did seem to have an overwhelming fear of needles, the consultant did not feel sure that the patient was incapable of weighing the risks and benefits of treatment. Rather, he felt that it was possible that the patient's value system was simply such that she weighed them differently than he would.

Questions

(1) Should the role of the consultant be to facilitate badly needed treatment by acceding to the obstetricians' request, or should the consultant cling to his opinion that the patient could be judged competent, even if that course results in the death of the patient and fetus? Are there other courses of action that might get the psychiatrist consultant "off the hook"? Are these "ethical"?

(2) Do you agree with the consultant that this patient is competent to refuse treatment? What criteria would you use for determining competency in this case? Do they differ from the criteria that you would use to establish competency in mental health settings? (See the cases in Chapter I.)

(3) Are there circumstances in which even a competent patient might legitimately be compelled to undergo treatment? Is this one of those situations? Can you think of others? Would you expect any of the philosopher consultants in Chapter 3 to support treatment over the patient's objections?

(4) What role do the rights of the fetus play in your approach to this situation? Can the fetus be said to have rights that are superior to the mother's?

(5) If the patient's family (husband and mother) were unanimous in either supporting the patient's or the obstetrician's position, would your reasoning change? What if the family splits in its support?

(6) Assume that the consultant writes the note that was requested and that induction of labor takes place over the patient's objections. A healthy infant is delivered, and the mother does fine in the postdelivery period. What recourse, if any, should the patient have against the obstetricians? Against the psychiatric consultant? Was she harmed in any way deserving of compensation? Did the physicians behave in any way deserving punishment? If so, what kind of punishment?

(7) Would your answer to question 6 change if a premature, nonviable infant is delivered? What if the reason for the prematurity is that the patient gave a misleading conception history in order to conceal the fact that conception occurred during the husband's absence?

VI

RELIGION AND MENTAL
HEALTH TREATMENT

PSYCHOSIS AND RELIGION

A conflict between the right to free exercise of religion and concern
about self-harm.

The patient was a 30-year-old, single man from India who was raised
as a Muslim. He had been hospitalized three times in the past year;
this admission was occasioned when he assaulted a passerby. At the time,
the patient was under the influence of a psychotic delusion that he was a
secret agent whose cover had been betrayed by his therapist.

Upon his admission, the patient refused medication on the ground
that he was a Christian Scientist. The surprised resident learned that
the patient had, while psychotic on his last admission, encountered
a Christian Science practitioner who was visiting the ward and decided to join the Christian Science Church. Consultation with the
practitioner raised the question of the extent to which the patient's
choice of Christian Science should be seen as a free choice, especially
since the practitioner did not view the patient as a true Christian
Scientist. On the other hand, the patient, although delusional, was
able to cite chapter and verse of Christian Science literature in support
of his drug refusal. The dilemma facing the resident was whether
this patient's religious choice was suspect because of his concurrent
delusional state, and thus whether his drug refusal based on this
choice was competent.

Questions

(1) The First Amendment gives us a right to freedom of religion. Would
this right be violated if this patient were forced to take medication?

(2) Is competence a prerequisite for extending a right?

(3) Using risk-benefit language, how would you make the argument for treating or not treating? You may assume that the benefit of treating is cure of the psychosis. The risk of treating is that various side effects may occur, including lasting and disabling movement disorders.

(4) How would you phrase the argument for either treating or not treating in terms of a language of "rights"?

(5) In questioning the competence of the patient's religious choice is the staff violating the patient's right to religious freedom? Is the question irrelevant, since religious choice is based on faith, which is beyond questions of competence?

(6) To be accorded appropriate weight, should a person's religious belief require the certification of an official practitioner? Specifically, should the clinicians in this case feel free to treat this patient's belief as delusional because the Christian Science practitioner sees the patient as "not a true Christian Scientist"?

ILLUSION OR TRUTH

Challenging religious beliefs in the interest of therapy.

The patient was a 30-year-old woman with a 6-year history of paranoid schizophrenia. Her father was an orthodox Jew, her mother a Protestant. Before she first became ill, she converted to orthodox Judaism.

The patient's hospitalizations would be precipitated by her refusal to eat, withdrawal, and finally catatonia, a condition in which she remained immobile for long periods of time. When she began to recover, she would not stay to participate in her treatment but would instead seek shelter in the orthodox Jewish community. On one of these occasions, when the patient went to Israel, she attempted suicide.

A senior clinician who began to work with the patient was confronted with the patient's use of Judaism in a self-defeating manner as a defense against serious engagement in treatment. The clinician also wondered whether the patient's use of Judaism in this manner, as well as her rigid orthodoxy, reflected unresolved issues regarding her father that the patient found too painful to face.

When, making no progress, the senior clinician had to terminate treatment the patient decompensated again. She entered the hospital, began to recover, and again began to retreat to the shelter of a supportive orthodox Jewish community. The new clinician doubted whether the patient would truly be helped by facing the "truth" that what she was holding on to was her father rather than Judaism. The dilemma facing the new clinician was whether to continue to confront the patient in therapy about the driving force for her religious focus or whether to try to help her make it as useful for herself as possible.

Questions

(1) Compare this case to three other cases: "Getting Better to Die" (Chapter IX), "Psychosis and Religion" (Chapter VI), and "The Right to Feel Good" (Chapter I). How is this case similar to and different from those cases?

(2) How valuable is the realization of the truth about one's self? To what lengths should a clinician go in order to promote this value?

(3) The patient's use of religion had been labeled a "defense," a "fixation," a mechanism to avoid something painful. Do patients have a right to such defenses? Would your answer differ if these defenses are working? If this patient was an involuntary one?

(4) Can one ever ethically justify a clinician's withholding from a patient an essential truth about that patient's condition? Under what circumstances?

(5) Is competence to give informed consent an issue here? If it is, how can the patient consent to receiving the truth about herself if she does not know ahead of time what the "risks and benefits" of such knowledge are? How can one relate to the patient the risks and benefits of such knowledge without conveying to the patient the knowledge itself?

(6) When discharged from the hospital, the patient repeatedly returned to a supportive religious community. If "curing" her of religious beliefs meant the loss of this source of support, would that affect your decision as to the proper approach to her treatment?

(7) Can there be childish and mature forms of religious belief and piety? Driven and autonomous ones? Can one avoid judging the nature of this patient's religious belief but continue to treat her?

BELIEFS UNTO DEATH

How should psychiatric staff treat patients whose religious beliefs cause others grave harm?

A 55-year-old female was said to have encouraged two other women to go on a 35-day fast (without food or water) that culminated in their deaths. She is a fundamentalist believer who states that she had turned her life over to God about 8 years earlier, and that she had a mystical or magical feeling as she made the decision. She says that God had commanded her to do certain things. Because of her new belief she claims that she was able to give up alcohol, depression, and some other unsavory aspects of her previous life. Since then she has been preaching the word of God. She says that she goes into churches and talks with many people when invited. But she denies having any followers or that she was the "teacher" of the two deceased women, as newspaper articles about their deaths had indicated.

She was admitted to a psychiatric unit, having signed herself in voluntarily after being brought there involuntarily from another hospital. Her husband ordered an ambulance to come for her because she had embarked upon a 40-day fast with no eating and no drinking. Her understanding of the fast was that she was following the command of God, and that God had told her that this was the way to bring salvation to her husband, who is a nonbeliever and who does not follow God's commands. According to her, God told her (directly and not through a hallucinated voice) that if she completed this fast her husband would achieve salvation. Apparently, after 35 days into the fast, the husband became concerned and she was brought to the first hospital. The patient denied any problems from the fast, indicating that she was somewhat slowed down. But she reported no difficulty in doing her work. Some of this seemed rather unlikely, in that survival without water for the length of time that she claimed would be unprecedented. She claims that she lost about 16 or 17 lb. during the fast but now she is up to 111 lb. Her normal weight is 116 lb.

She indicates that she was willing to come to the psychiatric unit because she knew it was God's will that she do so. But now, after 5 days, she wants to go home.

She is nonpsychotic and nondelusional in any conventional sense, although she firmly believes in what she tells the staff about her religious beliefs. She denies that her thought might be broadcast; she also denies having visual or auditory hallucinations, hearing voices, and the like. She seems to think rather clearly, consistent with the notion that God communicates to her, gives her commands, and rewards her appropriately. She has now decided that God no longer wants her to fast, that the fast should be ended at 35 days. Her thinking is reminiscent in part of the problems of cognitive dissonance; that is, she structures the facts in such a way as to preserve her belief system. She says that all she wants is to be left alone.

Questions

(1) Is this woman a "danger" to society?

(2) If so, should the staff attempt to have her confined for evaluation for a longer period than she wants?

(3) If she were likely to resume or repeat her fast, on orders from God, but not likely to involve others, would your answers change?

(4) Should the beliefs that encouraged two persons to die and that present a possible future danger to her be accepted as religious or challenged as possibly pathological? What if she had 500 followers? What if she were the head of an established 55,000 member religious organization?

(5) What are the dangers in attempting to distinguish between legitimate and pathological religious beliefs?

(6) What are the values we practice when we honor a patient's request to be "left alone"? Can this be a conflicted wish? What would we ask our ethical consultants in Chapter 3?

VII

ALLOCATION OF RESOURCES

"DO NOT RESUSCITATE" FOR THE LIVING

The responsibilities of staff and society to a deinstitutionalized patient, at an acute psychiatric facility.

The patient is a 50-year-old man with a diagnosis of mental retardation and a concomitant depression, as well as epilepsy. He has been an inpatient for the last three years at a community mental health center (CMHC), to which he was transferred from a large state hospital. He was the illegitimate child of alcoholic parents and has been a ward of the state since he was 3. Since that move two nursing home placements have been attempted, neither of which lasted longer than a month. According to the latest treatment plan, the patient requires services and training in the following problem areas: retardation and depression, personal hygiene, need for a citizen advocate to ensure availability of services, routine medical and psychological evaluations, grooming, eating, weight loss, chronic obstructive lung disease, seizure and movement disorder, obsessive concerns with death, a tendency toward masturbatory self-stimulation in public settings, the need to increase production rate at work, functional academic training, skills for self-preservation in society, learning of social skills, dentures, home placement.

The patient's transfer to the mental health center was part of a plan by the state's department of mental health to close down several units at the state hospital and to deinstitutionalize a number of patients. The review team in charge of this process of transfer determined that this patient and another had the greatest potential of all for development. A treatment plan was drawn up by the staff of the CMHC's developmental disabilities unit. The plan has as its goal residential placement in the community; the patient considered the transfer on that premise. Staff must now deal with the issue of the effort they must make to equip the patient for a move into the community.

Questions

(1) In ethical terms how would you characterize the responsibilities of society to this patient?

(2) What are the CMHC staff's duties to this patient?

(3) How would your answer to question 2 be influenced by the fact that (a) the CMHC's resources are limited, (b) other patients are present who would benefit to a greater degree, and (c) other patients are present who would have a better prognosis?

(4) In relation to the CMHC staff's duties noted above, how should the patient's behavior influence them? The patient's prognosis?

(5) Under what circumstances, if any, may a faculty "give up" on a patient with a nonterminal illness? Is the obligation to attempt to treat a limitless one? How, ethically, can limits be placed on therapeutic efforts?

(6) In what sense can this process of asking the above questions be helpful or harmful to the clinical care of this patient?

ONLY FOLLOWING ORDERS

Opposing superiors when harm to a patient is at issue.

The patient is a 56-year-old woman with a 20-year history of psychiatric illness, which manifested itself at times as a depressed state, at times as a paranoid, psychotic state. For the past few years, between her hospitalizations, she has lived in a nursing home. Before being hospitalized the patient stopped her neuroleptic medications, began withdrawing, and refused to eat. Indeed, this particular psychiatric hospitalization was preceded by a 40-lb. weight loss, a breakup with her boyfriend, and evidence of a psychotic thought process manifesting itself as the delusional belief that she was being poisoned.

For the first week the patient refused food, stating that hospital food was poisoned, and thus continued to lose weight; she also continued to refuse medication. Her new treating physician consulted with the senior supervising physician, and both agreed that the patient's continued psychotic refusal of food was putting her at risk of death. Since prolonged treatment could not be administered without a formal finding of incompetency and consent of a guardian, an emergency guardianship was applied for and obtained. Then, the patient was given neuroleptic medication by injection, the order being written as a "chemical restraint." This was the term used to describe medication being given in the face of a patient's refusal when there existed an imminent risk of harm to either the patient's self or to someone else.

The patient responded to this approach by becoming less openly psychotic, beginning to eat, accepting her medications, and beginning to form a relationship with her new therapist. She continued to improve to the point that the application for guardianship was withdrawn.

Three weeks later it was time for the therapist to go on vacation. In the past, under these circumstances, this patient would have continued on the locked unit until her therapist returned, as all staff agreed she would benefit from continuing in a holding environment, given the fragile connection she had reestablished with the treating institution. However, now that the hospital had undergone a reorganization, the number of beds on the Acute Unit had been sharply curtailed. As a result, conditions there had become dangerous because of overcrowding.

At a meeting of the senior staff it was decided that the least sick patient had to be discharged to lower the census immediately. The subject patient was chosen. The resident therapist was asked to write the order. However, he felt that other patients could be discharged more appropriately, and that his patient was being put at high risk of serious harm. After discussing this with the senior staff, he was overruled. He was told he had the choice of either discharging the patient himself or having it done by the administration.

Questions

(1) If you were the clinician, would you share this dilemma with the patient? If so, how would you do it? Why?
(2) What ethical justifications permit the resident to disobey the orders of his superiors?

(3) What level of risk to the patient should the resident accept before feeling justified in refusing to write the order? What other actions can the resident take?

(4) Under what circumstances should a junior trainee (the resident in this case) accept the validity of his own perceptions and resign, rather than follow orders?

(5) Under what circumstances should the senior staff who disagree respect the resident's decision and just write the order for him? Under what circumstances should a resident in that situation be fired?

(6) What are the sources of different perceptions of risk to the patient? To the Acute Unit as a whole? How should the senior staff's view of these risks be weighed against the resident's views?

(7) What approaches would you use in balancing the risks from discharge to the *individual* patient versus the risks from overcrowding to the patients on the Acute Unit *collectively*?

(8) To what extent can the struggle between the resident and his superior be considered a reenactment of the earlier struggle between patient and resident? What clinical issues and values must be explicitly addressed?

ADMISSION MISTAKES, DISCHARGE DILEMMAS

How should staff handle patients admitted too easily, who then do not want to leave?

A 45-year-old woman with a long psychiatric history was admitted to a psychiatric unit. Her complaints on admission were somewhat vague, but she came voluntarily, apparently seeking food and shelter. Utilization review concluded that this was an inappropriate admission, and shortly afterward the staff began to arrange discharge plans. The patient says that she wants to go to another state hospital, but the staff cannot transfer her there automatically. She spent some time talking to a representative from a mental health center that would need to evaluate her prior to transfer there. The center would not guarantee that they would send her to the state hospital. Apparently she has a long history of sabotaging a variety of discharge and community plans that have been made for her. Some attempt was made to contact her sister and brother-in-law, who initially said that they would pick her up and help her achieve some discharge plans, but they later reneged, saying that they did not want to get stuck with her either. There is a strong feeling on the ward that she should be discharged immediately, but she does not want to go.

The patient has about $6 to her name, enough for her to get to the mental health center by bus. She presents as a rotund, smiling, middle-aged female, difficult to follow at times. She sits quietly. She indicates that she would like to leave the hospital today and go to the state hospital. When confronted with the fact that staff can send her to the mental health center, but cannot guarantee admission to the hospital, she says she does not want to leave, that she has no place to go, that she needs a husband, that she is without emotional support.

Questions

(1) Does the decision (perhaps wrong) to admit this person to the psychiatric unit place obligations on the staff not to discharge her quickly?

(2) What are the ethical implications of admission decisions influencing subsequent therapeutic and discharge decisions?

(3) What are the obligations of hospitals and psychiatric staff to patients like this who cannot cope, but are not dangerous to self or others? What are society's obligations?

(4) Should financial considerations influence this judgment?

(5) If she objects to discharge, should she be forcefully ejected? If so, what responsibilities for follow-up will the hospital have?

(6) What action should be taken if the psychiatric unit were filled to capacity and there were an emergency admission waiting?

(7) How would each of the four ethical consultants in Chapter 3 advise you to pursue the process of inquiring into what is the "right" decision?

VIII

RESEARCH

WILLING SUBJECTS, QUESTIONABLE COMPETENCE

How should staff deal with patients willing to take part in low-risk experiments, but whose competence to consent is in doubt?

A psychologist is caring for an elderly woman inpatient with severe memory impairment, from whom he would like to obtain consent to do a diagnostic research protocol. The protocol itself is non-invasive and includes only sleep studies, neuropsychological testing, and EEG with evoked potentials. The patient appears to understand each component of the research, as well as the requests in general that she participate in research. However, she does not retain memory of any of this for more than a few minutes. It is not clear whether, when all of it is explained together, she retains the memory of the first part before the explanation of the last part is completed. Nonetheless she has been willing to go along. There is no family involved with her, but she does have a close friend. She has never been formally adjudicated incompetent. She was admitted to the hospital on a voluntary basis.

Questions

(1) How does the patient's memory impairment affect the giving of informed consent in this case?

(2) How meaningful ethically is the value of obtaining informed consent here?

(3) If you think it has little value, have you an alternative way of bringing patients like this into experiments?

(4) In this case, does the low risk of the experiment make a difference in the decision to admit her to the test?

(5) What if it were more risky? Would that change your reasoning, or the procedure that you would follow?

(6) If the patient were suffering from terminal carcinoma, would there be a change in the level of risk that you would find tolerable for the patient to assume without a meaningful informed consent?

(7) Suppose that the patient has a history of altruism, including an organ donor card that she had signed years before her illness. Should this make any difference? Discuss your answer from the standpoint of a "best interest" (decisions based on the best judgment of the decider) and a "substituted judgment" (decisions reflecting what the patient might have done) model of decision making for incompetent patients.

(8) What role, if any, should her friend play in this process? Should her friend be consulted and her approval obtained before allowing the patient in the experiment?

(9) Given this woman's mental state, should she have been allowed to consent to voluntary hospitalization, even if the laws of this jurisdiction do not explicitly require competent consent for admission?

WHEN SCIENCE AND PATIENT NEEDS CONFLICT

Should investigators who gain confidential information in the course of an experiment use it against the wishes of the subject?

As part of his thesis work, a graduate student is doing a follow-up study on patients who are not committed at hearings. At 30 days after the hearing, he is contacting the patients and asking to interview them, using a number of measures to determine their current status.

In this context, he went one night to speak with a 23-year-old single woman who was discharged to the care of her mother and father approximately a month before. He found her mute, withdrawn, practically catatonic, capable of giving only one verbal response in the hour and a half that he was there, and smiling inappropriately at the television set as he attempted to talk to her. Her mother reported that her weight, which had been 105 lb. (she is 5 ft. 7 in. tall) had dropped to 86 lb. over the last several weeks. The student found that both her mother and her father were significantly disorganized and had long psychiatric histories. Her mother said, "All she needs is a job." There are no other immediate family members involved. The graduate student thinks that the patient is desperately in need of hospitalization and that, in fact, she would qualify under a legal order for involuntary confinement as seriously impaired and in imminent danger. He struggles with the question of what to do about this information.

Note the methodology of his study and the way he obtains consent. He generally calls the patients or their families about the time that he wants to follow up on them, telling them of his dissertation topic and trying to arrange an appointment.

At the time of this encounter, he had tried to call the patient for several days at her boyfriend's house, where she was living. Although the boyfriend's son would answer the phone, the patient would not. He spoke with the patient's mother during that period, who had originally told him where the patient was. In a later call to the mother, she told him the patient was at home and invited him over to talk with her.

He never obtained the patient's consent to the encounter, but the mother was willing to sign the separate consent form that he had for the family. On the consent form, he assures the family that the information that he receives will be held confidential, elaborating only that their names will not appear on his forms. The consent form does not state what will be done with the information and does not mention whether it will ever be used as the basis for a patient's commitment. The student pays the family and the patient a total of $20 for their time.

The student recently completed a report on the performance of a unit whose lawyers represent mental patients at commitment hearings. The tone of the report and its conclusions were extremely critical of those lawyers who promoted the "best interests of the patients" rather than arguing as vigorously as possible for their clients' "rights."

Questions

(1) How does one weigh ethically the value to be attached to the privacy of the patient and the confidentiality of the communication given the investigator against the interest in protecting the patient from harm?

(2) Which is a better way to reason, to use the "rights of the patient" or the "best interests of the patient" as the yardstick?

(3) Under what circumstances should investigators use information obtained during research in the interest of therapy?

(4) Are investigators obliged to serve the needs of subjects when in the course of an experiment they obtain information that may benefit the subject?

(5) What would you do?

(6) Would your answer change if the patient revealed that she is planning to kill her mother?

(7) If you were on the research committee that reviewed this protocol, how would you have structured the procedure by which informed consent for the interview was obtained? Describe a model process and illustrate with a model consent form, stating how, with whom, and when it would be used.

(8) Would any of the philosopher consultants in Chapter 3 be of use in justifying the ethical value of research?

DETECTING CRIMES WHILE DOING RESEARCH

A conflict of research confidentiality, therapeutic benefit, and the social good.

A child psychologist has been working on research at a neuropsychiatric assessment center. The service gives comprehensive neurological, psychiatric, medical, and educational assessments to juvenile delinquents referred by Juvenile Court. He is now starting a pilot follow-up study of the first 50 children who were assessed 2 years ago, in order to obtain enough data to support a grant application for a more detailed study. He is looking at the court records to check on legal involvement, the history of subsequent placements, their social functioning, and whatever else he can find. He would now like to approach these 50 individuals directly to give them mental status examinations. He has the approval of the Juvenile Court for the study and the support of the administrators at his center.

The psychologist had come to the United States about 2 years ago and was not familiar with recent developments in this country on the ethics of clinical research. He had not considered whether and how consent would be obtained. His research advisor reviewed ethical issues that were raised by his study. These included: (1) The risk of provoking anxiety, if not paranoia, among juveniles who have been out of contact with the center and perhaps the juvenile justice system for at least 2 years, about who was keeping track of them and how the data that were collected at the center might be used in the future; (2) the risk of increasing their anxiety and the anxiety of their families by bringing up material and episodes that may lie buried in the family's mental attic of a time that was in all likelihood traumatic for them; (3) the possibility that by doing mental status assessments, he would raise the issue in the minds of the juveniles that perhaps they might be mentally ill, that they were selected for study because their assessment at the center revealed some sort of mental illness, and even if no signs of mental illness had developed until now they might appear in the future; (4) the question of what he would do with the information gathered if he discovered that any of the patients were mentally ill and in need of treatment (it is not unlikely that a number of these children are psychotic and not currently in treatment, and some of them might even be so psychotic as to be committable); (5) the question of what to do with information that he might gain about crimes in which these children have participated, are participating, or intend to participate in the future; and (6) the issue of who gives consent for entry into the study (most of the children that he will follow up will be between 16 and 17 years of age and familial consent would appear to be necessary in addition to their own consent).

Questions

(1) In each of the above questions, what are the values at stake and in conflict?

(2) How would you deal with the ethical dilemmas raised by each of the above considerations?

(3) Should this study be done?

(4) How would you obtain consent? What wording would you use? From whom would you seek consent? Would you approach the individuals for informed consent alone, or in the presence of their parents?

(5) Would your answers change if the children were younger than 12 years old? Younger than 10?

IX

MENTAL HEALTH AND
MEDICAL ILLNESS

READING A CLOSED BOOK

How far must staff go in treating a patient who declines therapy?

M r. Y. is a 30-year-old man with prune-belly syndrome (a serious metabolic disorder) and secondary chronic renal failure. The patient was born out of wedlock, abandoned by his mother. Prune-belly syndrome was evident at birth. The patient was placed in a foster home, but the multiple medical problems of his condition necessitated admission to a state hospital, where he remained for approximately 15 years before transfer to a state school for the retarded.

The patient's renal problems have been chronic, severe, recurrent, and nearly untreatable. He had had nine separate major urologic surgical procedures, including total removal of a left kidney at the age of 7. His course has been complicated by numerous infections, imbalances of his electrolytes and metabolism, hypertension, and general progressive deterioration. In the several years before admission, he developed a left brain hemorrhage after a fall, which required surgery; he then required the same procedure after another fall a year later. Regrettably, a seizure disorder developed (which is often the case in such injuries) and the patient is now on anticonvulsant medication. The patient was recently begun on chronic hemodialysis because of the functional failure of his kidney. However, the course of his treatment has been extremely stormy with the patient being both despondent and uncooperative. Repeated shunts to connect the patient to the dialysis machine have had to be placed in the patient's blood vessels because he frequently manipulates the shunt tubing and has had recurrent infections around the shunt site.

Within the past 6 months the patient has attempted to throw objects and food into the dialysis machine. He indicated he doesn't like his dialysis treatments and wishes they would stop. In turn the dialysis team has questioned the continued efficacy of treating this patient in the light of his refusal and his tendency to be an extreme management problem and a disruptive force on the otherwise tranquil dialysis unit. Furthermore, the patient's emotional disorder has been characterized by aggressive behavior. Ten years earlier, the patient became severely assaultive and violent, and had to be committed to a state hospital. Shortly afterward he attempted suicide by jumping out of a window and was again committed. When admitted to general hospitals, he was described as having many temper tantrums and being prone to powerful swings of mood. On several occasions he broke hospital windows, pulled out his catheters and smeared them in feces. Attempts at behavior modification, pharmacological interventions, and other management approaches have been notably unsuccessful.

Questions

(1) Are patients in general free of ethical obligations? If no, what are the patient's ethical obligations in this case? If yes, what is the basis for that view?

(2) How do you justify continuing treatment in this case? How do you justify discontinuing treatment?

(3) According to the case as presented, the patient "indicates" that he does not like dialysis and wants it to stop. What would be your basis for accepting this as a valid statement? For rejecting it?

(4) The two standards in use for surrogate decision making at this time are the best-interest standard, according to which one determines the best decision without necessarily referring to the patient's perspective, and the substituted judgment standard, which would have the therapist glean the basis for choosing from the life of the patient. Discuss their differences, and which you would use in this case of essentially lifetime incompetence.

(5) What is the ethical argument for and against considering a patient's intelligence as a factor in the amount of resources society should expend in providing medical treatment? What about other mental

or physical attributes? Where would you draw the line as to what attributes (e.g., "beauty," "religion") should under no circumstances be considered? Apply your reasoning about the above to this case.

THE "CATCH-22" SYNDROME

Trying to treat patients who keep changing their mind.

The patient is a woman in her 40s who presented with adenocarcinoma of the breast which, although first diagnosed 4 years before admission, was never treated because of the patient's refusal. During the previous year, after an extensive workup, the breast mass was found to be approximately the size of a softball, with diffuse local invasion but, surprisingly, as yet there was no evidence of spread throughout the body. During the admission to a psychiatric hospital for evaluation of her mental status, the patient first denied the existence of the mass and refused physical examination. After discharge the patient was referred back to her medical hospital for follow-up, but never returned (as was her usual pattern).

Two months later the patient was brought to the hospital for court evaluation on the charge of arson, apparently stemming from her attempt to "keep warm" by setting a small fire in her building. During the admission, a concerted, prolonged effort to develop an alliance became possible and the patient finally consented to have a physical examination, which revealed the mass described above and the presence of enlarged auxiliary lymph nodes – an indicator of the beginning of systemic spread of her cancer. The need for appropriate medical-surgical intervention at this point became far more pressing, and attempts were made to engage the patient in reaching a proper decision regarding her care. With time the patient's profound denial abated and she consented to the treatment. As the day approached for her transfer to the appropriate facility, however, she became more despondent; the denial, now psychotic in extent, resurfaced, and finally the patient escaped. After about 10 days the patient "happened" to be walking by the hospital and was easily convinced to return to the ward. Since then two guardians have been appointed.

The first proved uncooperative and ambivalent about the decision-making duties, and thus the appointment of the second was necessitated in the interest of the patient's receiving care. On at least one subsequent occasion this behavior has recurred: The "catch-22" for this patient is that she is willing to accept the reality of her illness and consent to having treatment as long as the treatment is not imminent; but paradoxically and regrettably, as treatment *becomes* imminent, the patient's competence to consent is vitiated by the return of her psychosis-induced decompensation. In other words, she is only competent to consent to treatment when she won't be having it; when she is about to have it, she becomes incompetent to consent to it.

Questions

(1) On ethical grounds, should the patient's refusal of treatment have been honored or overridden during the first admission? What about after the second admission, with the spread of the cancer?

(2) Is ambivalence of the sort that this patient exhibits an appropriate general warrant to act on the patient's behalf *without* the patient's wholehearted agreement? As a related question, is ambivalence of this severity tantamount to incompetence?

(3) One school of thought might argue that the resolution of the problem is simply to ask, "What does the patient really want?" What are the limitations and problems with this approach? What other approaches might you recommend?

(4) What are the ethical problems with a patient whose decision-making capacity depends on the situation as it presents itself?

(5) Odysseus bound himself to the mast to avoid changing his mind, and in certain cultures the best man's job the night before the wedding is to get the groom sufficiently inebriated to prevent any last minute "cold feet" absconding. What about using such a mechanism in this case, e.g., giving the patient high doses of a minor tranquilizer? Would it make any difference whether the patient requested it? Use *both* patient autonomy and his or her best interest to argue for or against such an approach.

GETTING BETTER TO DIE

Should we use our medical skill to increase the awareness of a patient that death is near?

The patient is a woman in her 60s with an absolutely classical involutional depression: the serious depression that comes on in later life and is characterized by severe psychotic disturbance and somatic delusions (e.g., images of one's insides rotting). This troublesome affliction responds well to electroconvulsive therapy, which is 90 percent effective and highly safe in patients having this diagnosis. This particular case has a complicating factor, however; the patient also has been diagnosed as suffering from a severe carcinoma, systemwide in its spread, which has reached the stage of untreatability and signals death in the near future. The depression, however, is preventing the patient from having full awareness of this fact. In offering her electroconvulsive therapy, the staff members recognize that her mood may return to normal; the reality that she will *then* face is that of imminent death.

Questions

(1) Discuss the case in terms of the Hippocratic moral precept describing the doctor's task as being "to help or at least do no harm."

(2) The fact that this patient will die is the truth. Is helping this patient recognize the truth an ethical good?

(3) It could be argued that the patient has two illnesses, depression and cancer, and you are simply treating the treatable one. What ethical issues does this position obscure?

(4) Suppose, instead of the relatively safe electroconvulsive therapy, the only treatment available carried a significant degree of risk of shortening the patient's life (although it would cure the depression). Justify the use of this therapy. Justify nonuse of such a treatment.

(5) Analyze the same case supposing that resources for treatment are severely limited (the triage argument).

(6) In what sense is involving the patient in the decision-making process a clinical good? An ethical good?

(7) Compare your conclusions about this case with the situation in "The Right to Feel Good" (Chapter I).

X

MENTAL HEALTH AND CRIMINAL JUSTICE

ON PROBATION

The validity of a patient's consent to share medical data with legal
authorities.

The patient is a paranoid schizophrenic male in his 20s who was
first admitted several years ago by his mother after she found
him sitting in the kitchen at 3 a.m. with the gas jets on the stove
turned up full. The patient stated he turned the stove up to keep
warm and hadn't noticed the house being filled with gas fumes.

The patient had dropped out of school at the age of 16 and
experienced gradual withdrawal accompanied by poor concentration
and auditory hallucinations; he had spent most of the year prior to
his first admission alone in his room listening to music. In the past
2 years the patient has been admitted to the hospital eight times.
Typically, he would request admission because of hearing voices and
worrying about losing control. He would recompensate fairly rapidly, become involved in ward activities, then would deny that he
had any problems, sign a self-discharge paper, and leave the hospital.
Of these admissions, five have been voluntary, one civil involuntary,
and two based on court orders for seemingly impulsive criminal acts,
which tended to occur shortly after the patient stopped taking his
medication.

Most recently he threw a brick through a police car window and
was consequently sent by the court for psychiatric evaluation. The
hospital found him competent to stand trial and recommended further inpatient treatment and medications. He was placed on 1-year's
probation and now returns to the hospital, where he signs in vol-

untarily. Two days afterward he signs a request for release. Since the hospital had received no communication from the court as to the condition of his probation, staff request and receive the patient's permission to inform his probation officer of his actions. The probation officer hurries to the hospital and tells him that he cannot leave until the hospital team feels he is ready; moreover, if he does so against advice, he will be considered in violation of his probation and will go directly to jail. The patient then withdraws his request to leave.

Questions

(1) In what sense is this patient's present admission voluntary; in what sense involuntary?

(2) Discuss the elements of coercion given in the case, explicit and implicit. Can the inmate of a "total institution" ever give consent that is not coerced at some level? How should such consent be obtained and honored by the conscientious clinician? What are the implications of your answer for possibilities of research on such populations (which may represent their only future hope of help)?

(3) What are the ethical complications when psychiatric treatment is made a condition of parole?

(4) What is the validity of this patient's consent to have his confidentiality broken? To have this consent later used "against" his express wishes to leave the hospital? What should the clinician tell the patient to make this consent as informed as possible?

(5) Assume that at the very beginning of the admission the clinician had made a contract with the patient and with the parole officer, whereby the patient agreed at the outset that the parole officer would be notified of any pending discharge plans. Could such a contract be ethically valid? If this contract were made a *condition* of the admission, how should one regard the patient's later wish to "retract" the contract? What are the minimum conditions for such a "therapeutic contract" to be ethically valid? To be therapeutic?

(6) Would the violence of the crime of which the patient was convicted change your answer to any of the above questions?

DETECTIVE OR DOCTOR?

What, if any, are the obligations of mental health staff to aid police investigation of patients?

The patient is an unemployed man in his mid-30s who was admitted to a psychiatric hospital with the tentative diagnosis of schizophrenia.

Near the time of this admission, the hospital's continuing care division was notified by the landlady that the patient was causing difficulty in the apartment complex where he was living and that the police had been called. The patient had apparently followed a young woman into the laundry and made what were interpreted as sexually provocative comments. The woman was frightened and called the police, who interviewed the patient; the latter denied any wrongdoing, and no charges were filed.

The landlady, however, became concerned about the safety of her four children living on the premises and requested that the patient be removed. The hospital's continuing care division contacted the police and discovered that the patient had applied for a gun permit sometime earlier. In addition, the police had a record of charges against the patient, including breaking and entering, child molestation, violation of parole, kidnapping, rape, and assault with a deadly weapon. To further complicate matters, the patient had a younger stepbrother with exactly the same name to whom some or all of these charges might conceivably apply; although there was no mention of these charges in the patient's hospital record, it was known that he had once been a security guard and had carried a gun.

The patient was contacted by phone and asked to come to the clinic for an evaluation. He came that evening. He was asked to wait in the lobby while some details of the case were sorted out by telephone, but during this time, before the evaluation was finished, the patient left the hospital. On the grounds that the patient was a threat to others, the doctor in charge filed an involuntary commitment request, and the patient was returned to the hospital that same evening by the police. During this process the patient was hostile, violent, and uncooperative and had to be tended by security personnel and secluded. After release from the seclusion room, he was docile and cooperative and professed ignorance of any reason for his admission. He was not thought to be psychotic at any time.

The next day it was learned that the police had an outstanding warrant dating from 10 years earlier for the arrest of someone by the patient's name on a charge of molestation of a 15-year-old girl. In addition the patient had apparently been sentenced to a long stay in prison 3 years later for a charge of rape, kidnapping, and assault with a deadly weapon. The patient denied all of these charges against him.

To sort out this conflicting information, the police suggested that fingerprints be obtained. The patient agreed to fingerprinting by his physician on the inpatient unit after the situation was fully explained to him and after he gave his written consent. However, his resident physician did not consult anyone about this procedure. The prints confirmed that the police had a correct record of charges against him from 10 years ago but did not have a correct record of the subsequent charges.

Since there was an outstanding warrant for his arrest, the police requested that they be notified when he was to be discharged from the hospital. As there was now no specific psychiatric reason for keeping him in the hospital, the patient was discharged and taken for questioning by the police. He was invited to get in touch with his doctor after his legal status had been clarified so that outpatient therapy could be continued. The patient was released after several days and returned to his apartment but refused either to come to the outpatient department or to vacate his apartment. After several hearings the charges against him from several years ago were dropped. However, his neighbors continue to be frightened by his presence, and the situation remains unresolved.

Questions

(1) What confusions, from an ethical standpoint, are introduced when the therapist fingerprints the patient? For example, suppose the patient was thus found to have committed a serious, previously undetected crime?

(2) What is the significance of the patient's consent to this procedure?

(3) Suppose the patient told the therapist that some of the crimes attributed to his brother had in fact been committed by himself. What could be the ethical obligations of the therapist to the patient? To the police? To the landlady? To society at large? Which takes precedence? Under what circumstances?

(4) The patient in this case apparently discontinued treatment in part *because* the treatment staff "turned him over to the police." Discuss the ethical tension between the goals of treatment for the patient, protection for society, the fostering of justice, and cooperation with the police.

(5) Is this a case in which the patient's autonomy and the protection of

society come into conflict? The patient's autonomy and the therapist's autonomy? What would you have done and why? As the case unfolds, at what point, and with what question, would you ask for an "ethics" consultation or discussion?

THE THERAPIST AS POLICEMAN

Exploring therapeutic responsibility in police failures.

A 27-year-old male presents himself to the hospital emergency room seeking admission. He is well known to the personnel as a man with chronic paranoid schizophrenia, alcoholism and some antisocial traits. His history includes assaultiveness, multiple detoxifications, and much talk of violence, including statements on several occasions that he has killed people and been in a large number of fights. Over the years his therapists have assumed that these boasts were largely untrue.

The patient presents for admission drunk, asks jokingly if he has to hit the therapist to get admitted, but does not appear to be threatening. The therapist tries to arrange an admission for detoxification, but the facility refuses the patient.

Two days later the police call the therapist, saying that the patient has confessed to them that he murdered a man in a downtown hotel room. His complete confession includes descriptions of the room, the man's clothes, and the scene. Even so, the police express doubt about the patient's actual culpability since he could well have acquired the information through questions "on the street." They indicate that since they believe they have no grounds for holding him, they plan to discharge him to his mother's care and bring him back for questioning the next day.

During this conversation, the therapist shares his opinion that the patient is potentially dangerous and urges the police to hold him in jail or have him committed to a hospital; the police express reluctance to do this. The therapist worries about his own liability if the patient, released, harms someone, as – he reasons – the patient may well do to "prove" he is sick enough to be hospitalized. In his own heart he believes the patient did commit the murder.

After extensive consultation, the therapist decides to offer the patient voluntary hospitalization while the whole affair is sorted out.

Questions

(1) The therapist spontaneously related to the police his belief that the patient was dangerous. In whose interest might that statement have been made? Are there conflicts of interest here? What duties here are ethically owed the police? Owed the patient? Owed others?

(2) What considerations govern the therapist's obligations (in the matter of the alleged murder) to the patient? To society?

(3) Even if the police do not believe the patient, may or should the therapist act out of his own conviction that the patient did commit the murder? For example, should the therapist petition for the patient's commitment on the basis of a danger not recognized by the police?

(4) What considerations govern the offer for voluntary hospitalization to sort things out?

(5) Would your answers be different in the case of a planned as opposed to a completed murder? What if the alleged murder had occurred 10 years earlier?

(6) What general rules can you construct that would govern the relationship between the police and the mental health professions? How are their proper spheres of activity demarcated? What would be the effect of applying your rules in this case?

(7) Which of the above considerations would you share with the patient?

THE MENTAL HOSPITAL AS JAIL

The role of the hospital in the containment of "dangerous" persons.

A 30-year-old man seeks admission for fear that he may harm his common-law wife as he has been hitting her and losing his temper with her. He requests help for self-control. His history reveals many fights, and one conviction 4 years earlier of assault on a relative that put him in prison for 2 years; he is now on parole. He has deliberately avoided seeking help in his own area since he feels he is "too well known there," and that may prejudice his care. He is admitted, although it is not clear that his problem (a character disorder) will be helped by acute hospitalization, because of the evaluating clinician's fear that he may harm his wife.

After he is admitted, the security unit tells the staff that there is a warrant out for the patient's arrest on charges of statutory rape and assault on his own daughter. The security personnel state that they will notify the police that he has been admitted; no one seems to know if security has the patient's permission to do this. Later it is discovered that 3 days before admission the patient received a phone call warning him about charges being filed, and the patient left immediately "to get help."

Confronted with this information, the staff raise the following questions: Although the patient should probably be in some kind of confinement, should it be in a hospital? Is there anything a hospital can do for him at this point? Is the entire admission manipulative, a means to get away from the legal charges?

The patient refuses permission to contact his parole officer. The parole officer, however, calls the ward and asks to speak to the doctor, who urges the patient to grant consent to talk to him; the patient agrees. The parole officer asks how long the patient has been and will be in the hospital, since the parole officer plans to have him arrested. The doctor gives the date of the expected discharge and tells the parole officer about a plan to have the patient arrested as he leaves the ward. The patient is not told of this.

After the discharge, the arrest takes place as planned. The therapist later informs the parole officer of a threat the patient made against the officer; during the conversation the officer asks for more information about the patient. The therapist refuses this and several subsequent requests, not having obtained the patient's permission.

A letter from the patient, now in jail, arrives one month later, stating that he feels betrayed by the hospital on two grounds. First, he is upset about the arrest itself, for he feels he was "set up." Second, he is angered that the doctor mentioned how long he had been in the hospital, since this led to additional charges of violating parole, based on the length of time the patient had been out of his home county (a condition of his parole being that he could not be absent more than a short period of time).

Questions

(1) In this case, there is clearly tension between the risks to security posed by a potentially dangerous patient and the requirements of

confidentiality in the therapeutic setting. At what points does this tension become manifest? Comment on the decision made at each of the points, noting whether your response would differ from the doctor's in the case.

(2) What considerations do you think governed the therapist's warning to the parole officer about the threat? The therapist's urging the patient to permit communication with the parole officer? The decision to have the patient arrested off the ward? The patient not being told of this plan? Comment on the ethical tensions inherent in each of these decisions.

(3) What case could be made for the hospital staff refusing to acknowledge to anyone that the person was even a patient on the ward, regardless of the criminal charges?

(4) Are there any circumstances under which clinical staff, convinced that a patient is seeking to be admitted specifically to avoid or mitigate the effects of legal process, should participate (or collude) in this process?

(5) The fact that in this case "everyone feels responsible for what happened except the patient" is of clinical interest. Is it of ethical interest?

WHEN THE POLICE DICTATE THE TREATMENT

To what extent should a clinician allow a patient's treatment plan to be determined by requests from the criminal justice system?

A psychiatrist at an alcohol and drug abuse treatment center was contacted by a therapist at the center about a patient she had evaluated previously and referred for treatment. The patient was now suspected by the police of setting a series of fires that had terrorized the neighborhood in which the center was located. The police believed that the patient, who was on parole from a prison term for arson in another state, set the fires when he became drunk. Although they lacked sufficient evidence to arrest the patient, they were certain enough of his involvement to ask the psychiatrist to take immediate steps to make sure that he did not become drunk again and set more fires. Specifically, they requested that she start the patient on Antabuse, a medication that discourages patients from drinking as it induces a severe physiologic response following the consumption of alcohol; the response can be severe enough to cause death.

The psychiatrist believed, however, that this patient was not a good candidate for Antabuse because he was an active binge drinker who had showed little motivation to stop. She feared that if he were started on the medication, he might drink anyway and suffer life-threatening consequences. At the same time, she believed that the patient might benefit from inpatient detoxification, a course that she supported but he had been reluctant to accept.

The following day the patient himself appeared at the clinic requesting Antabuse. In the meantime, he had been called in by his parole officer and told that he was a prime suspect in the cases of arson; he had been informed that if he showed evidence of drug or alcohol use, his parole would be revoked and he would be sent back to prison to complete the remaining 13 years of his 20-year term. The psychiatrist refused to initiate Antabuse, but did urge the patient to enter a detoxification program voluntarily, as she had promised the police that she would. The patient refused at first, but after coaxing by the psychiatrist and his parole officer, agreed three days later.

After being admitted to the detoxification center, the patient was told that the parole officer had revoked his parole on the grounds that his entry into a detoxification program proved that he had been drinking, and this was contrary to the conditions of his parole. He was sent back to prison in the other state. The spate of fires ceased.

Questions

(1) Should the psychiatrist have agreed to the police request that she initiate treatment with Antabuse to protect the public in a very dangerous situation? What ethical principles are in conflict here?

(2) When the patient, fearful that he might lose his freedom as a result of his continued drinking, asked her to prescribe Antabuse for him, should she have done so at that point? What ethical principles are in conflict here?

(3) What is the relative balance between the psychiatrist's obligations to society, her patient, and her professional standards in such circumstances?

(4) In general, does society have the right to specify the kind of treatment that patients should receive to protect society? Does a patient's involvement with the criminal justice system affect that right? Consider in your response an exhibitionist who has been ordered to receive behavioral therapy as a condition of probation; a child molester who

is ordered to undergo treatment with hormones that will lower his sex drive; a spouse abuser who is required to enter an alcohol treatment program; a chronically psychotic schizophrenic, arrested repeatedly for disturbing the peace, who is ordered to accept antipsychotic medication; and a patient similar to the last one, except that he has no record of arrests.

(5) Consider the following variant: In another country a new treatment for alcoholism is developed – a long-acting form of Antabuse that can be injected and is efficacious for up to a year after injection. Under what conditions would you consider it ethical that a patient be mandated to receive such an injection? What if the intervention involved minor surgery to place a time-release reservoir in the abdominal cavity? Would it make a difference if the country in question had a totalitarian form of government?

(6) When a clinician believes that a form of treatment ordered by a court (e.g., as a condition of probation) is inappropriate for a particular patient but it is clear that unless the treatment is provided the patient will be returned to jail, should the clinician go along with the court's order? Does this depend on the possible risks of treatment? On its cost? On the amount of the clinician's time that the treatment will require? On whether the clinician believes the patient was innocent of the original charges?

(7) How would you characterize the parole officer's actions in having the patient's parole revoked? Would a clinician be justified in refusing to cooperate with this parole officer in the future? Even if the public safety were at stake?

(8) Under what circumstances would it be ethical for the clinician to initiate contact with the patient's legal aid attorney?

BIBLIOGRAPHY

This bibliography is divided into ten sections, each corresponding to the topical divisions of the cases presented. We hope these essays and books will help readers gain a broader view of the choices and problems raised in the cases.

I. Informed consent, competency, and involuntary treatment

Appelbaum, P. S., & Roth, L. H. (1981). Clinical issues in the assessment of competency. *American Journal of Psychiatry, 138*:1462–1467.

Bursztajn, H., Feinbloom, R. I., Hamm, R. M., & Brodsky, A. (1981). *Medical choices, medical chances: how patients, families, and physicians can cope with uncertainty.* New York: Delacourt/Seymour Lawrence.

Bursztajn, H. (1985). More law and less protection: "critogenesis," "legal iatrogenesis," and medical decision making. *Journal of Geriatric Psychiatry, 18*:143–153.

Doudera, A. E., & Swazey, J. P. (1982). *Refusing treatment in mental health institutions: Values in conflict.* Ann Arbor, MI: AUPHA Press.

Gutheil, T. G., & Appelbaum, P. S. (1982). *Clinical handbook of psychiatry and the law.* Chap. 5. New York: McGraw-Hill.

Michels, R. (1981). The right to refuse treatment: Ethical issues. *Hospital and Community Psychiatry, 32*:251–255.

President's Commission for the Study of Ethical Problems in Medicine and Biomedical and Behavioral Research. (1982). *Making health care decisions: The ethical and legal implications of informed consent in the patient–practitioner relationship: Vol. 1. Report.* Washington: U.S. Government Printing Office.

Rachlin, S. (Ed.). (1985). *Legal encroachment on psychiatric practice.* San Francisco: Jossey-Bass.

Roth, L. T., Appelbaum, P. S., Sallee, R., et al. (1982). The dilemma of denial in the assessment of competency to refuse treatment. *American Journal of Psychiatry, 139*:910–913.

Stone, A. A. (1982). Introduction to "Law and Psychiatry." In L. Grinspoon (Ed.), *Psychiatry 1982: The American Psychiatric Association annual review.* Washington, D.C.: American Psychiatric Press.

II. Confidentiality

Appelbaum, P. S. (1982). Confidentiality in psychiatric treatment. In L. Grinspoon. (Ed.), *Psychiatry 1982: The American Psychiatric Association annual review.* Washington, D.C.: American Psychiatric Press.

Beck, J.C. (1985). *The potentially violent patient and the Tarasoff decision in psychiatric practice.* Washington, D.C.: American Psychiatric Press.

DeKraai, M. B., & Sales, B. D. (1984). Confidential communications of psychotherapists. *Psychotherapy, 21*:293–318.

Stone, A. A. (1983). Sexual misconduct by psychiatrists: The ethical and clinical dilemma of confidentiality. *American Journal of Psychiatry, 140*:195–197.

Wulsin, L. R., Bursztajn, H., & Gutheil, T. G. (1983). Unexpected clinical features of the Tarasoff decision: The therapeutic alliance and the "duty to warn." *American Journal of Psychiatry, 140*:601–603.

III. Truth-telling

Billings, J. A. (1985). Sharing bad news. In Billings, *Outpatient management of advanced cancer.* Philadelphia: J. B. Lippincott.

Bok, S. (1978). *Lying: Moral Choice in Public and Private Life.* New York: Pantheon Books.

Bok, S. (1982). *Secrets.* New York: Pantheon Books.

Bursztajn, H. (1977). The role of a training protocol in formulating patient care instructions as to terminal care choices. *Journal of Medical Education, 52*:347–348.

Bursztajn, H., Hamm, R. M., Gutheil, T. G., & Brodsky, A. (1984). The decision analytic approach to medical malpractice law: formal proposals and informal synthesis. *Medical Decision Making, 4*:401–414.

Halleck, S. L. (1984). The assessment of responsibility in criminal law and psychiatric practice. In D. N. Weisstub (Ed.), *Law and Mental Health: International Perspectives.* Vol. 1. New York: Pergamon Press.

Novack, D. H., Freireich, E. J., & Vaisrub, S. (1979). Changes in physician's attitudes toward telling the cancer patient. *JAMA, 241*:897–900.

Reiser, S. J. (1980). Words as scapels: Transmitting evidence in the clinical dialogue. *Annals of Internal Medicine, 92*:837–842.

IV. Managing difficult patients

Adler, G. (1973). Hospital management of borderline patients. *American Journal of Psychiatry, 130*:32–35.

Bursztajn, H., et al. (1981). *Medical Choices, Medical Chances – How Patients, Families and Physicians Cope with Uncertainty.* New York: Delacorte/Seymour Lawrence.

Bursztajn, H., Gutheil, T. G., Hamm, R. M., & Broadsky, A. (1983). Subjective data and suicide assessment in the light of recent legal developments. Part 2: Clinical uses of legal standards in the interpretation of subjective data. *International Journal of Law and Psychiatry, 6*:331–350.

Bursztajn, H., Gutheil, T. G., & Cummins, B. (1986). Legal issues in patient psychiatry. In Sederer, L. I. (Ed.), *Inpatient Psychiatry.* Baltimore: Williams and Wilkins.

Cohen, R. E., & Grinspoon, L. (1963). Limit setting as a corrective ego experience. *Archives of General Psychiatry, 8*:90–95.

Gralnick, A. (1979). The management of character disorders in a hospital setting. *American Journal of Psychotherapy, 33*:44–66.

Groves, J. E. (1978). Taking care of the hateful patient. *New England Journal of Medicine, 298*: 883–887.

Gutheil, T. G. (1982). On the therapy in clinical administration. *Psychiatric Quarterly, 54*:3–25.

Gutheil, T. G. (1985). Medicolegal pitfalls in the treatment of borderline patients. *American Journal of Psychiatry, 142*:1, 9–14.

Gutheil, T. G., & Havens, L. L. (1979). The therapeutic alliance: Contemporary meanings and confusions. *International Review of Psychoanalysis, 6*:467–481.

Gutheil, T. G., & Rivinus, T. M. (1977). The cost of window breaking. *Psychiatric Annals, 7*(2):47–51.

Johansen, K. H. (1983). The impact of patients with chronic character pathology on the hospital inpatient unit. *Hospital and Community Psychiatry, 34*:842–846.

Stone, A. A. (1984). *Psychiatry and morality: Essays and analysis.* Washington, D.C.: American Psychiatric Press.

Talbot, E., & Miller, S. C. (1966). The struggle to create a sane society in the psychiatric hospital. *Psychiatry, 29*: 165–171.

V. Parents and children

See also References at the end of Chapter 3.

Giovannoni, J. M., & Becerra, R. M. (1979). *Defining child abuse.* New York: The Free Press.

Weithorn, L. A., & Cambell, S. B. (1982). The competancy of children and adolscents to make informed consent decisions. *Child Development, 53*:1589–1598.

Winnicot, D. W. (1987). *Babies and their mothers.* Reading, MA: Addison-Wesley.

VI. Religion and mental health treatment

Favazza, A. R. (1982). Modern Christian healing of mental illness. *American Journal of Psychiatry, 139*:728–735.

Peteet, J. R. (1981). Issues in the treatment of religious patients. *American Journal of Psychotherapy, 35*:559–564.

Spero, M. H. (1981). Counter-transference in religious therapists of religious patients. *American Journal of Psychotherapy, 35*:565–575.

Spero, M. H. (1983). Religious patients in psychotherapy: Comments on Mester and Klein "The young Jewish revivalist." *British Journal of Medical Psychology, 56*:287–291.

Mester, R., & Klein, H. (1981). The young Jewish revivalist: A therapist's dilemma. *British Journal of Medical Psychology, 54*:299–306.

VII. Allocation of resources

Childress, James F. (1970). "Who shall live when not all can live," *Soundings, 53*:339–355.

Daniels, Norman (1985). *Just health care*. New York: Cambridge University Press.

Goldman, H. H., Pincus, H. A., Taube, C. A., & Revier, D. A. (1984). Prospective payment for psychiatric hospitalization: Questions and issues. *Hospital and Community Psychiatry, 35*:460–464.

Halleck, S. (1981). Covert values in the treatment of psychosis. *American Journal of Psychology, 35*:173–186.

Hiatt, H. H. (1975). Protecting the medical commons: Who is responsible? *New England Journal of Medicine, 293*:235–241.

Hamm, R. M., Clark, J. A., & Bursztajn, H. (1984). Psychiatrists' throny judgments: describing and improving decision making processes. *Medical Decision Making, 4*:425–447.

Reiser, S. J., Anbar, M. (eds.): (1984). *The machine at the bedside: Strategies for using technology in patient care*. New York: Cambridge University Press.

VIII. Research

Appelbaum, P. S., & Roth, L. H. (1982). Competency to consent to research: A psychiatric overview. *Archives of General Psychiatry, 39*:951–958.

"Final Report of the Tuskegee Syphilis Study Ad Hoc Advisory Panel." (1973). Washington, D.C.: U.S. Public Health Service. Reprinted in S. J. Reiser, A. J. Dyck, and W. J. Curran (Eds.). (1977). *Ethics in medicine: Historical perspectives and contemporary concerns*. Cambridge: MIT Press.

Golby, S. (1971). Experiments at the Willowbrook State School. *The Lancet, 1*:749.

Roth, L. H., Appelbaum, P. S., Lidz, C. W., Benson, P., & Winslade, W. J. (in press). Informed consent in psychiatric research. In A. Brooks, & B. J. Winick (Eds.), *Mental health law: Developments in the 1980's*. New York: Guilford Press.

IX. Mental health and medical illness

Annas, G. (1982). Forced Caesarians: The most unkindest cut of all. *Hastings Center Report, 12*(3):16–17, 45.

Appelbaum, P. S., & Roth, L. H. (1982). Treatment refusal in medical hospitals. In President's Commission for the Study of Ethical Problems in Medicine and Biomedical and Behavioral Research, *Making Health Care Decisions, Vol. 2*. Appendix. Washington, D.C.: Government Printing Office.

Bursztajn, H., & Barsky, A. J. (1985). Facilitating patient acceptance of a psychiatric referral. *Archives of Internal Medicine, 45*:73–75.

Bursztajn, H., Gutheil, T. G., Warren, M. J., & Brodsky, A. (1986). Depression, self-love, time, and the "right" to suicide. *General Hospital Psychiatry, 8*:91–95.

Bursztajn, H. (1986). Ethicogenesis. *General Hospital Psychiatry, 8*:422–424.

Leiberman, J. R., Mazor, M., Chaim, W., et al. (1979). The fetal right to live. *Obstetrics and Gynecology, 53*:515–517.

President's Commission for the Study of Ethical Problems in Medicine and Biomedical and Behavioral Research. (1983). *Deciding to forgo life-sustaining treatment*. Washington, D.C.: Government Printing Office.

X. Mental health and criminal justice

Appelbaum, P. S. (1984). The expansion of liability for patients' violent acts. *Hospital and Community Psychiatry, 35*:13–14.

Appelbaum, P. S. (1984). Hospitalization of the dangerous patient: Legal pressures and clinical responses. *Bulletin of the American Academy of Psychiatry and the Law, 12*:323–329.

Freud, S. (1916). Some character types met in psychoanalytic work; "the exceptions." Reprinted in *The complete psychological works of Sigmund Freud*, standard edition, 14:311–314. London: Hogarth Press, 1957.

Halleck, S. (1971). *Psychiatry and the dilemmas of crime*. Berkeley, CA: University of California Press.

Vaillant, G. E. (1975). Sociopathy as human process. *Archives of General Psychiatry, 32*:178–183.

INDEX